The Sweet Life

How (and Why) to Live Free of Processed Sugars ... and Love it!

Content, Recipes, and Photos By
Dr. Brandie Gowey, NMD

Foreword By
Laura Brummels,
Social Thinking Therapist
and Speech Pathologist

Edited By
Charlotte Fox

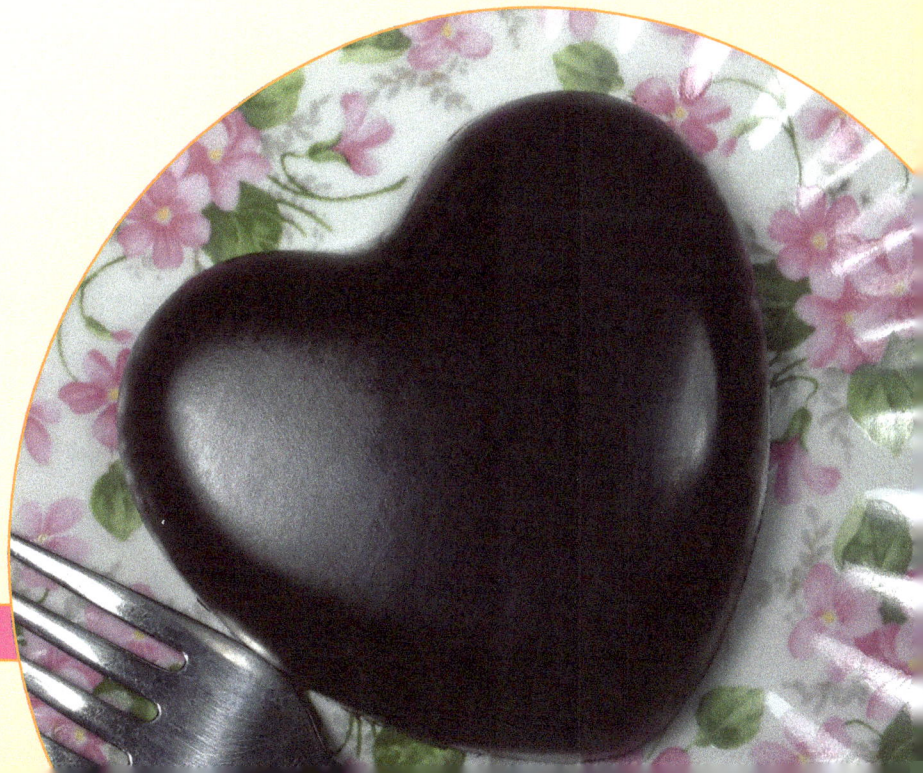

The Sweet Life

**How (and Why)
to Live Free of Processed Sugars
... and Love It!**

Published by
DR. DNA Press
Flagstaff, AZ

Printed in the United States of America

ISBN 978-09861850-1-4

Cover and Book Design by
Andi Kleinman

Proceeds from the sale of this book benefit
medical research at DR. DNA Clinic.
Learn more at *goweyresearchgroup.com*.

Dedicated to my friend Ian Ross, who believed in me from the day we met, long before I ever considered going to medical school.

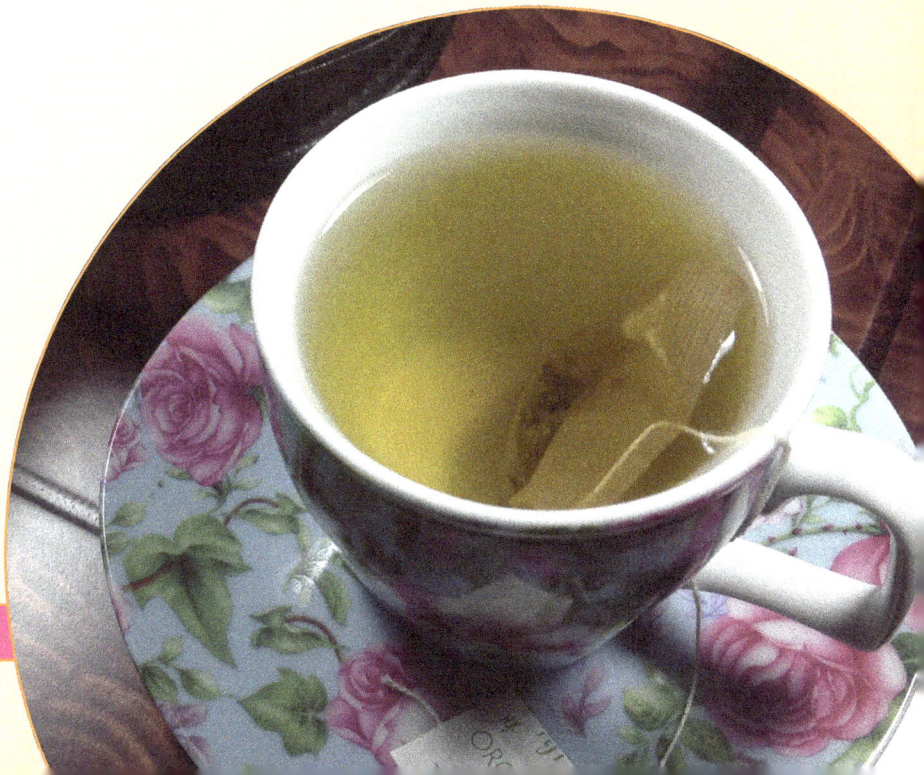

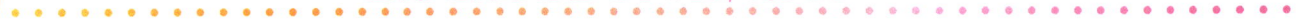

Table of Contents

FOREWORD

I resonate with this book because I've had personal experience with both processed foods and sugar. Eating sugary foods causes me to feel a range of emotions from hyperactivity to anxiety or lethargy. Or, I will feel hungrier and overeat.

I have witnessed similar behaviors in my children and the students I work with. I can recall an incident with one of my online students. He's 15 years old and has a diagnosis of high functioning autism. He signed into our 50-minute session on time, and ready to work. 5 minutes into the session, his mom brought him a can of soda and a bag of chips. About 20–25 minutes later, I noticed his eye gaze shifted from me to the window in the kitchen, and then to the other room, and his cat etc. I spent the remainder of the session helping him refocus his attention to the task at hand. I see this a lot in my practice. I feel it is the sugar causing this. My students who abstain from sugars do not exhibit this extreme of behavior, they are more calm and focused, and it only takes a short period of time to see a difference.

Statistically speaking, the average CHILD consumes 49 pounds of sugar a year.

When I read this statistic I immediately thought, "that's not me, or my kids, we're healthy", but as I started looking more closely at the foods in our home —bread, applesauce, yogurt, chips and even salsa, I was surprised to learn that I have been extremely mislead. Sugar really is, "EVERYWHERE", and it hides. This, as a result, which you will find out, is a public health issue. Dr. Gowey goes into great detail in her book about how and why processed foods and sugar create significant problems for the immune system, and that, over time, create common medical conditions such as cancer, anxiety, ADD/ADHD, chronic pain, and insomnia. There is no coincidence that these conditions plaque our society.

The contents in this book are so shocking, startling and real! I encourage you to read this book very carefully and thoughtfully, and with a mind that's open to having your dietary beliefs challenged. I hope she inspires you to not only examine the labels of the foods that read "natural" and "healthy", but also look deeper into how sugary foods make you feel.

The recipes she provides are both simple and delicious. Some of our favorites include her Chicken Nuggets, soups and broths, Bunless Burger, Breakfast Bake, smoothies, Yummy Beets and salads.

Digest this book, and you'll truly LIVE THE SWEET LIFE!

LAURA BRUMMELS,
Social Thinking Therapist and Speech Pathologist

Journal Your Thoughts

Record Your Progress

Note Your Recipes

PREFACE

This book started out as a reference guide as to the impact sugar has on your immune system. After sending the draft for editing, the feedback I received was that this book was "too technical". At that point I changed gears in an effort to make this book more palpable. I added recipes, made the information simpler and pulled a good deal of information. But after months of editing, I realized I was not doing anyone any favors by trying to make the subject of this book easier.

You need to avoid processed foods (sugars) as much as you possibly can. They create unpredictable chaos within your body and prevent healing (Xuan et al. 2014). There is absolutely *no* way to avoid chronic disease, cancer, autoimmune disease, or any other challenging health condition by eating sugar.

Our grocery store shelves are full of sugar, its "everywhere" as my patients say. But as you read through this book, you will gain an understanding that living without sugar is incredibly necessary.

Avoiding sugar is the one thing you can do to prevent most illnesses. Get your children in the no-sugar habit and you will see how both you and your family are happier and healthier, sleep better, and have greater energy or focus. If you don't heed the warning your immune system is giving you via adverse symptoms created by consuming sugars, then I am afraid you are living on borrowed time: at some point a deleterious health condition will manifest. However, many chronic diseases and conditions are preventable and based on choices you make in your lifestyle.

Introduction

When was your first experience with processed sugar? Do you remember? Or has sugar been such an integral part of your life that you can't actually recall "a first"?

My first experience with sugar came when I was 4 or 5 years old. My dad tells the story of buying me a Snickers® candy bar while at a convenience store, and giving me a small piece. He said that as soon as I got it in my mouth, my eyes got huge! After chewing and swallowing the little piece of chocolate, I turned to him with angry, accusing eyes, and said, "You've been holding out on me, haven't you, dad?"

Therapist Laura Brummels says that sugar has become our reward. We are taught at a young age that if we "eat our vegetables" we can have our cookie. I see this way of thinking deeply ingrained in my patients' lives: if "I lose just a little bit of weight, I can have that ice cream. I deserve it!"

Sugar is in almost every processed food on the shelf, from soups to chips, to yogurts and teas. We start giving it to our children at an early age, eat it while we are pregnant, when we are stressed, and we eat it as though it is one of the food groups (Halloran 1994).

We love our glucose, honey, corn syrup, fructose, agave syrup, table sugar, maple syrup, and manufactured sugars such as Splenda®. We eat products called "KIND" bars because the marketing on the package assures us they are "KIND":

> Do the KIND Thing—for your body, your taste buds, and the world!® KIND is a brand of delicious, all natural foods made from ingredients you can see and pronounce.® At KIND, we do things differently and try to avoid false compromises. Instead of "or" we say "and." Healthy and tasty, convenient and wholesome, economically sustainable and socially impactful. A study by the Yale–Griffin Prevention Research Center indicates that eating two KIND bars a day helps prevent weight gain.

"KIND" bars tend to contain a few types of processed sugar in each bar, including honey and glucose. My patients who abstain from all forms of processed/packaged sugar find that just one bite of one of these bars start to "almost instantly" make them feel very ill. From one of my patients:

> After abstaining from all forms of processed sugars for months, I decided I deserved a little treat. I picked a KIND bar because the label said it was "all natural". Later that day, however, I started to feel awful. At 11:30 PM I awoke from sleep feeling angry, depressed, and all my joints were in extreme pain. I started to beat myself up mentally about just about everything in my life. I just knew it had to be the sugar because I had not had any in months. My symptoms continued for hours during the night, and finally into the early morning hours I fell back to sleep. I woke feeling upset and still

in pain. I had no idea even the "natural" sugars are just as processed as the rest, and can make me feel just as bad.

Sugars on the market, whether labeled as "natural" or not, are all processed. This includes honey and maple syrup unless you are purchasing direct from the producer a product that has not been pasteurized, for if it has been processed in any way, it looses so much of its nutrients.

And, if it looses its nutrients, it becomes a detriment to the immune system, something **that hurts the immune system rather than heal it.**

As of 2014, Americans ate on average 22 teaspoons of sugar per day (authoritynutrition.com).

Beginning in the 20th century, the world population of 1.6 billion consumed 8 million tons of sugar.

Today at population of 7 billion, the world consumes 165 million tons of sugar (sueden.com) and the average child consumes 49 pounds of sugar per year (parents.com).

From USDA.gov, per capita consumption of table sugar and corn sweeteners (such as high fructose corn syrup) increased 43 pounds (39%) between 1950 and 2000.

There are 4 grams of sugar in a level teaspoon. To give you an idea of some sugars in popular foods and beverages, see the following list:

❥ Starbucks® Vanilla Bean Crème Frappe® = 57 grams of sugar

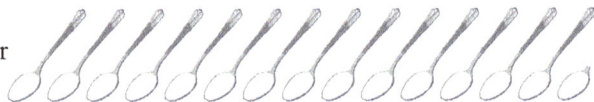

❥ McDonalds® Mocha Frappe = 71 grams of sugar

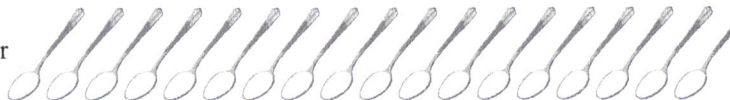

❥ Cold Stone® Creamery Ghirardelli Chocolate ice cream = 26.7 grams of sugar

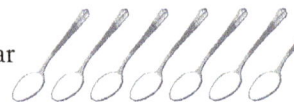

❥ Mars® Milky Way Bar, 2 oz = 35 grams of sugar

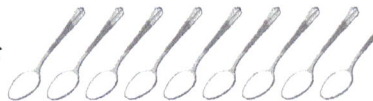

❥ Glutino® Gluten-free Pretzels, 24 pretzels = 24 grams of sugar

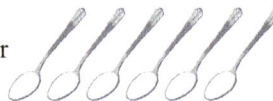

Foods such as these elevate the blood sugar. If the blood sugar elevates (even transiently), it can create problems for the immune system. There are 4 main ways your blood sugars can elevate:

1. Dietary Exposure

2. Stress

3. Medications

4. Environmental Toxins (Malekir et al. 2013)

Unfortunately, over time the rise in blood sugars can create just about any kind of medical condition. Here are some examples:

- ADD/Hyperactivity in Children
- Allergies
- Anxiety
- Arthritis
- Autoimmune Diseases
- Cancer
- Chronic Pain Disorders
- Depression
- Fatigue
- Fibromyalgia
- Insomnia
- Irritable Bowel Syndrome
- Mood Disorders

This book is about the 4 ways your blood sugar can elevate and the subsequent effect on your immune system. This information is provided to help you understand the importance of sugar abstinence.

Of the 4 reasons your blood sugars can elevate, changing your diet is the one you have the most control over.

You can live a health-filled, happy life WITHOUT SUGAR!

No! You don't actually need that ice cream right before bed. What you *really need* is a nice cup of tea, WITHOUT SUGAR!

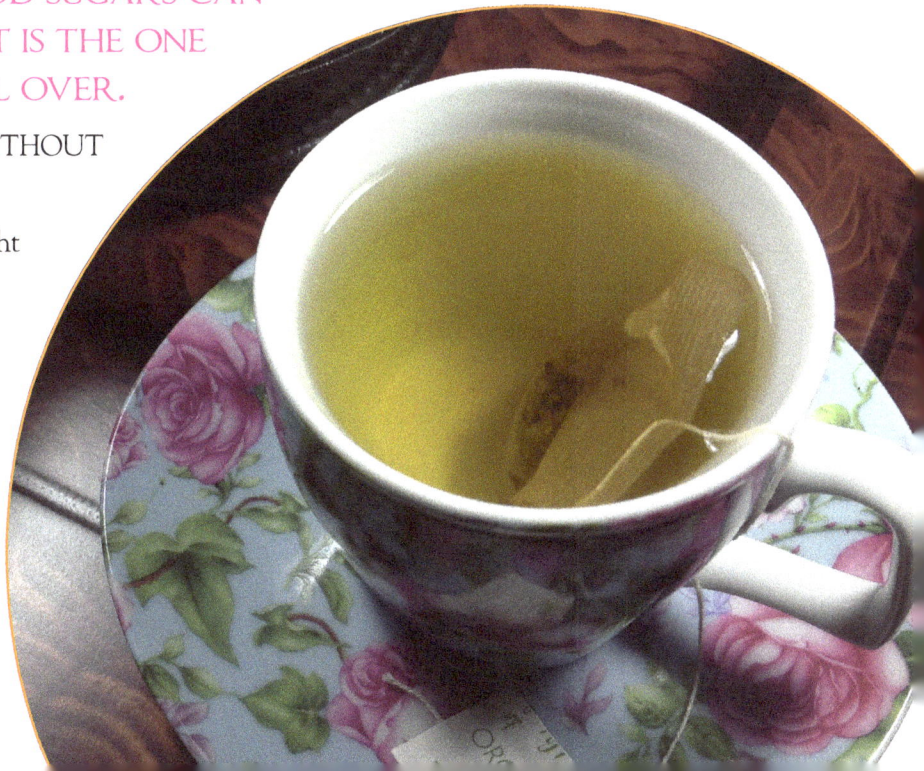

The chapters in Part One explore the four ways your blood sugar can elevate:

Dietary Exposures

Stress

Medications

Environmental Toxins

Part One

4 Ways Blood Sugars Elevate & How They Affect Your Immune System

Breakfast Bake

1 pound Italian Sausage

4 Potatoes, peeled and shredded

4 Eggs

1 pkg Spinach, fresh (or frozen, unthawed)

4–5 baby Tomatoes

Cook the sausage thoroughly in a thin layer of water. In a 9–inch baking dish, place a layer of the potatoes on the bottom and cover with the sausage and drippings. In a separate bowl, whip together the eggs, spinach and baby tomatoes and pour over the potato and meat layers. Bake at 350 degrees for one hour or until the eggs are fully cooked.

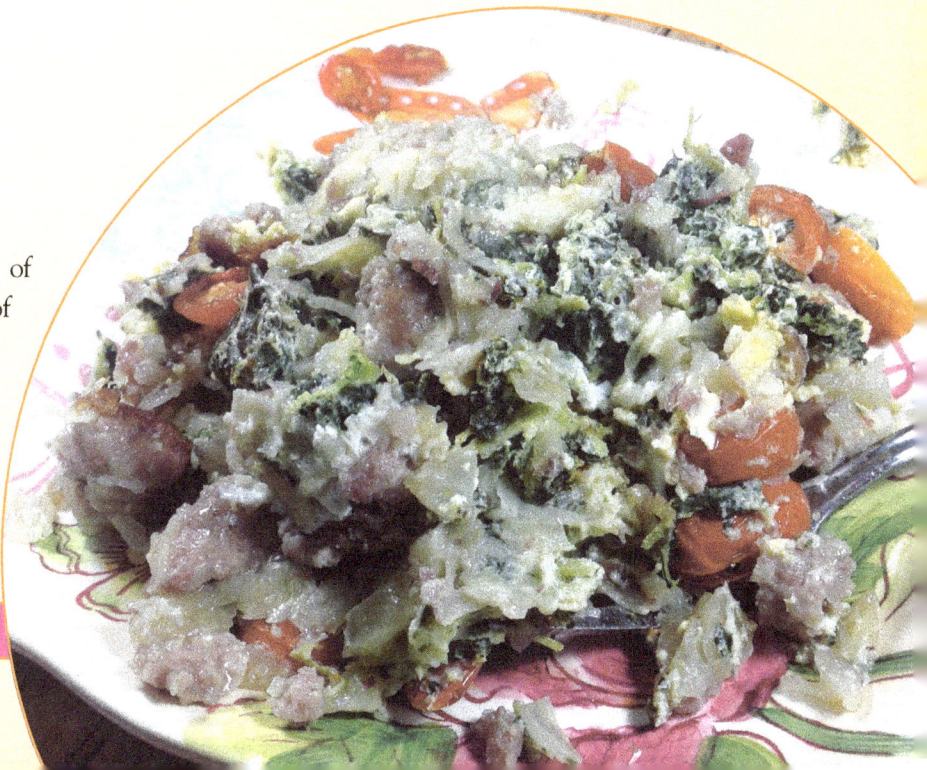

CHAPTER 1

BLOOD SUGAR LEVELS
&
DIETARY EXPOSURES

FRUIT CONCENTRATE TOPPING

2 Apples, peeled and chunked

1, 10 oz pkg Raspberries

Combine in a saucepan and simmer, stirring until liquid is evaporated and fruit is thickened. Serve over potato pancakes.

POTATO PANCAKES

5-6 medium Red Potatoes, shredded

2 Eggs

¼ Onion, chopped

Salt and Pepper to taste

Mix all ingredients together and form into flat cakes. Cook in a skillet in butter or coconut oil until brown on both sides. Great served with Fruit Concentrate Topping.

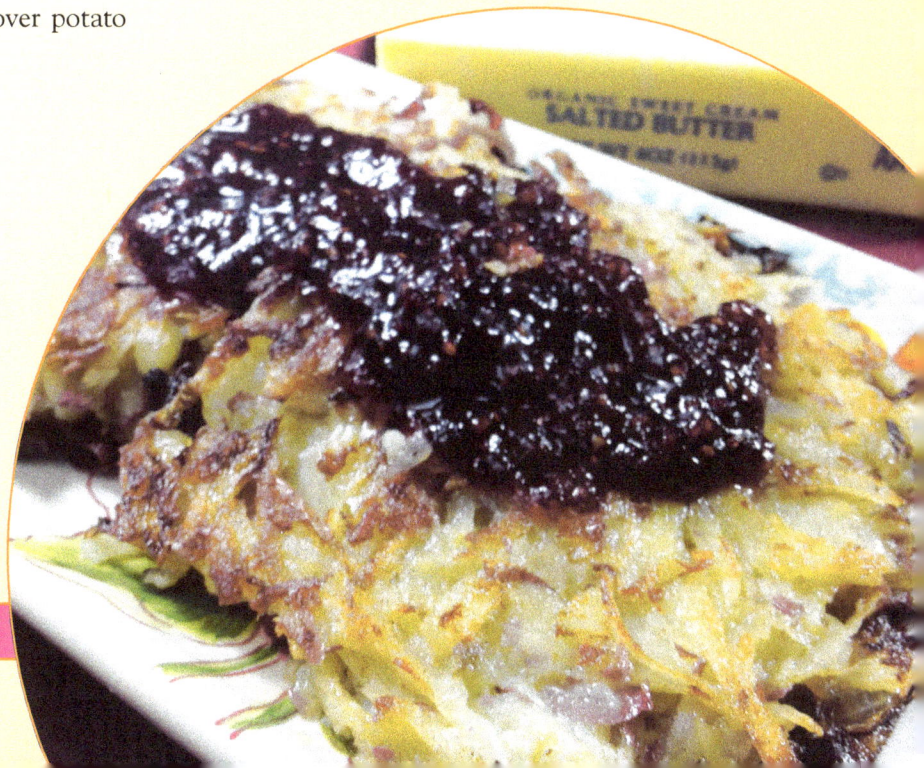

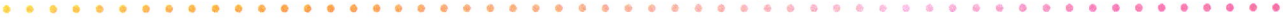

Chapter 1

Blood Sugar Levels & Dietary Exposures

As a society, we consume much more sugar than we realize. Sugars are added to just about any food you can think of! To get an idea of how the sugar can create problems, I would like to give you an idea of how it affects *you*.

I would like to challenge you to do a little experiment. Start by taking a good look at your diet. What are the most common foods you eat? Look at labels and examine where you are getting added processed sugars from, and make a list of the top 10 foods you are eating that have sugar in them:

1. _____
2. _____
3. _____
4. _____
5. _____

6. _____
7. _____
8. _____
9. _____
10. _____

Now, eliminate all forms of these foods and any other processed sugar and foods *for at least 3 months*. This means looking at labels closely because sugar is added to a lot of foods, including gluten-free snacks, pastas, soups, salad dressings, beverages, or restaurant foods. I also would like you to avoid all processed grains, including breads, pastas, crackers, or any other food that is sent through a mill to produce. Focus on eating berries (especially organic) and fatty foods (such as olives or nut butters without sugar added) if you have a sugar craving. The berries (because they're high in antioxidants) will help keep your blood sugar levels even, as will the good fats.

Now that you have analyzed your diet and avoided all processed sugars *for at least 3 months* go ahead and have many processed and sugar-rich foods as you would like over the course of the day, then list here any symptoms you experienced. Most people notice symptoms within a few minutes to an hour of eating something with sugar, so pay close attention to how you feel. List some of your symptoms on the following page.

1. _____ 4. _____

2. _____ 5. _____

3. _____ 6. _____

Depending on your sensitivity level, overall disease processes, and genetics, you should experience a change to your symptoms or feelings with and without sugar. Sugar is the most powerful immune-changing "chemical" I have ever experienced, so much so that I have never had a patient tell me that sugar abstinence did not help reduce negative symptoms, no matter how subtle or drastic symptoms are.

Once you have eliminated processed sugar for 3 months, try the same experiment with processed foods (i.e. breads, pasta) and then have a whole pizza and see how different you feel! Sluggish? Short temper? It is because the foods are processed!

_____

_____

_____

_____

_____

_____

_____

_____

_____

_____

CHAPTER 2

BLOOD SUGAR LEVELS
&
STRESS

FRESH OATMEAL

There really is no reason to purchase oats that have already been cooked and have sugar added. The steel-cut or uncooked oats really are the best tasting, and do not take that long to cook. I like to cook my oats in filtered water, and add fresh berries right before serving. I also like to add a dash of cinnamon for some extra spice.

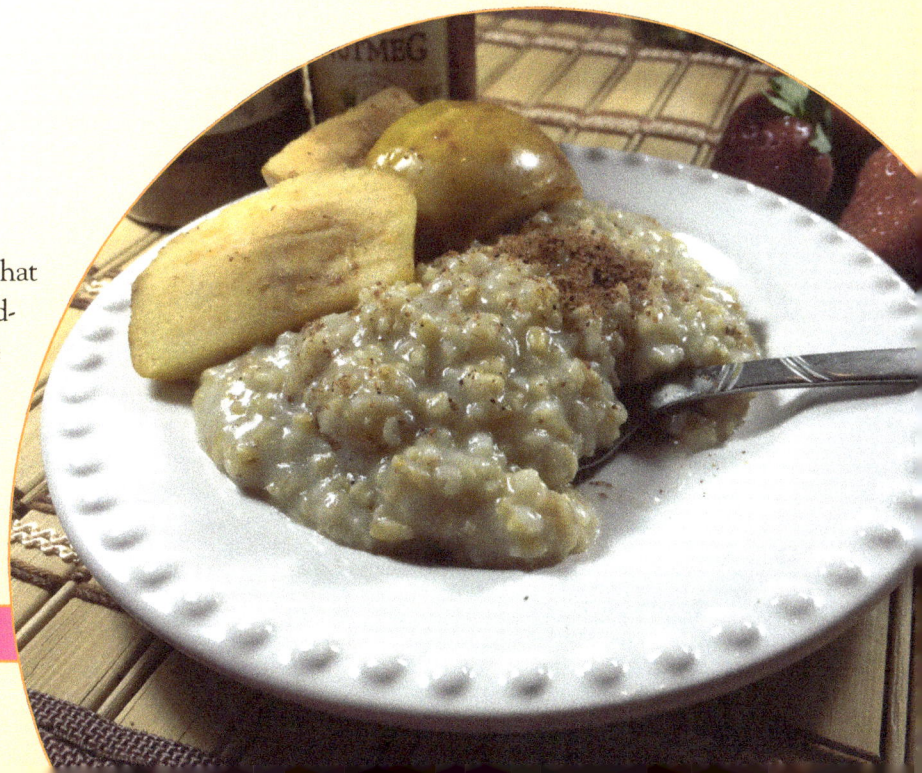

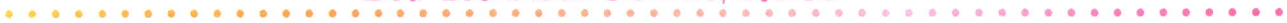

CHAPTER 2

BLOOD SUGAR LEVELS & STRESS

Stress increases the levels of a hormone called cortisol. Cortisol sends a signal to the liver that has an effect of increasing blood sugar levels. This is a natural process that is supposed to happen to help us through stressful times. From an evolutionary perspective, an elevated cortisol under duress would have kept blood sugars high while we may not have been able to eat.

An un-stressed cortisol has a natural rhythm: it is higher in the morning, has a few peaks and valleys throughout the day, and then drops at night. These shifts create changes in your blood sugar throughout the day. This is what the normal cortisol rhythm looks like:

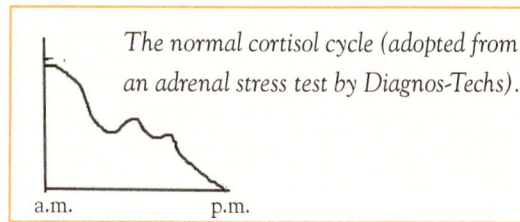

The normal cortisol cycle (adopted from an adrenal stress test by Diagnos-Techs).

In comparison, this is what a "stressed" cortisol rhythm looks like:

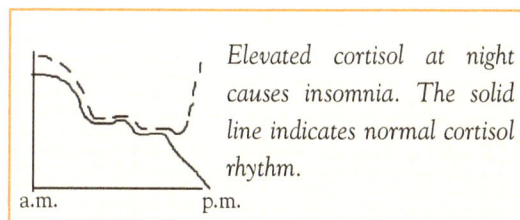

Elevated cortisol at night causes insomnia. The solid line indicates normal cortisol rhythm.

However, if the stressor does not decrease, or if your reaction to the stressor does not change, cortisol can remain elevated, either all day or at times during the day. This is especially the case for those who struggle with insomnia. Elevated cortisol at night is what usually keeps them up.

If the cortisol is elevated, **blood sugars stay high** because of the signal that is automatically sent to the liver to release stores of sugar.

Coconut Milk Soup

1 can Coconut Milk

Water

1 tbsp Curry Powder

½ cup Onion, chopped

½ cup Green Beans, diced

½ cup Broccoli, chopped

½ cup Carrots, diced

2 small Red Potatoes, diced

Pinch of Salt

½ cup Rice, cooked

Open the can of coconut milk and pour into a soup pot. Fill the can with water and add to the milk. Add all ingredients and allow to simmer on low until the veggies are cooked all the way through. Add ½ cup cooked rice at the last 5 minutes of heating.

Variation: Add cooked tofu chunks or chicken. Serve with fresh greens on top, such as watercress or bean sprouts. I also like to make this soup with just chopped onions and potatoes. With the curry spice added this makes for a very nourishing soup. Sometimes I also add ½ cup spinach at the last few minutes of cooking. The frozen spinach works well for this.

Chapter 3

Blood Sugar Levels & Medications

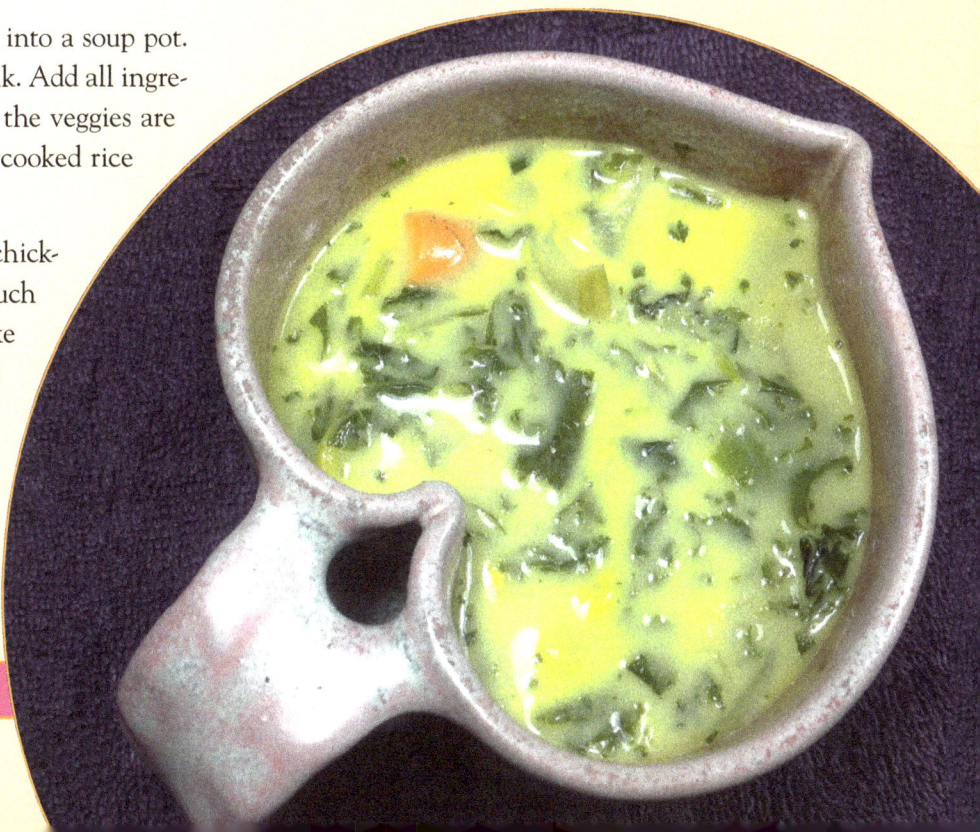

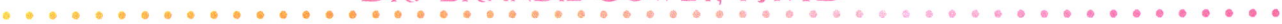

Chapter 3

Blood Sugar Levels & Medications

There are a handful of commonly prescribed medications that can increase blood sugars. Here are some of the most common types of medications. Do any of these sound familiar (webmd.com and everydayhealth.com)?

Anti-depressants	Barbiturates	Estrogens
Anti-inflammatories	Corticosteroids	Lithium
Anti-psychotics	Decongestants	Oral Contraceptives
Aspirin	Diuretics	

While some of these medications may be necessary to extend life, many are over-used, over-prescribed, or abused. When considering your medical needs, choose your medications wisely and with careful counsel by your physician.

SIMPLE SMOOTHIE

4–6 Organic Oranges, freshly juiced

2, 8–12 oz bags of Organic Strawberries

1 cup Water

Blend together (the Ninja® blender works great!) and enjoy.

SIMPLE SMOOTHIE, No. 2

4–6 Oranges, freshly juiced

2 pkgs. frozen Organic Strawberries (or berries of choice)

½ cup Kale or Chard

1 cup Water

Pop everything into a blender and blend until smooth.

Variation: Add a splash of Fresh Lemon Juice and a tbsp of Coconut Oil (or any Omega Oil for the added benefit of an essential fatty acid).

SMOOTHIE POPSICLES

1, 10 oz bag Berries, frozen

½ cup Coconut Milk

Blend and freeze into popsicles (I found popsicle sticks at Michaels).

Variation: Use fresh squeezed Orange Juice instead of the berry/coconut milk combination.

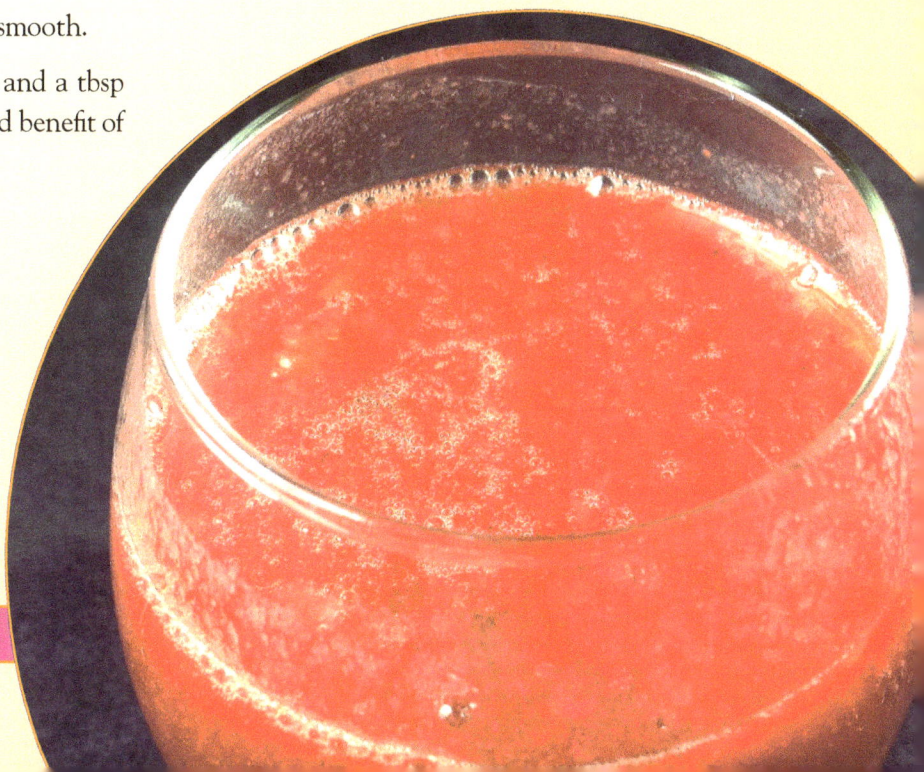

CHAPTER 4

BLOOD SUGAR LEVELS & ENVIRONMENTAL TOXINS

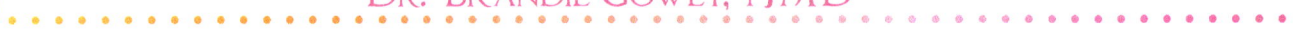

CHAPTER 4

BLOOD SUGAR LEVELS & ENVIRONMENTAL TOXINS

There are number of chemicals (such as pesticides) that are known to raise blood sugar levels. Farmers who handle these chemicals are particularly prone to the development of high blood sugar levels:

> *About 25 million agricultural workers in the developing world suffer from at least one episode of poisoning every year, mainly by anticholinesterase–like organophosphates (OPs)… the exposed farmers showed higher fasting blood glucose… anxiety/insomnia and severe depression were also significantly higher in the farmers than in controls. Farmers showed clinical symptoms of eczema, saliva secretion, fatigue, headache, sweating, abdominal pain, nausea, superior distal muscle weakness, inferior distal muscle weakness, inferior proximal muscle weakness, breath muscle weakness, hand tingling, foot tingling, euphoria, polyuria, miosis, dyspnoea, bradycardia, and rhinorrhoea, which all significantly correlated with the number of working years. These findings indicate that farmers who work with OPs are prone to…diabetes* (Malekir et al. 2013).

You eat these chemicals, especially when you do not buy organic foods. Antioxidant-rich foods help protect your DNA from damage (Mullner et al. 2013), but if you are eating non-organic foods with the chemicals on them, your blood sugar will be affected. This counters the effects of eating the antioxidant foods.

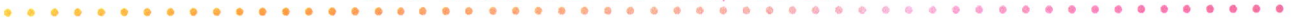

Your body is very conservative with energy. If your blood sugars elevate and you don't need these sugars for immediate energy, then the cells of your body will do one of two things with the excess calories:

... either they will adhere the sugar to a red blood cell (called a "hemoglobin A1c", or HgA1c)

... or they will convert the sugar into a fat.

The problem with both is that your immune system will be affected in adverse ways.

The chapters in Part Two review these two processes.

PART TWO

WHAT DOES YOUR BODY DO WITH EXCESS BLOOD SUGARS?

POPCORN

Popcorn Kernals

Coconut Oil

Butter, melted

Salt

Nutritional Yeast

Layer the bottom of a small (lidded) cook pan with the coconut oil (or you can air pop your popcorn). Once the oil has melted, sprinkle the kernals on the bottom of the pan. Cover the pan and place on medium heat. Allow the popcorn to pop fully and remove from heat. Add melted butter, salt and nutritional yeast to taste.

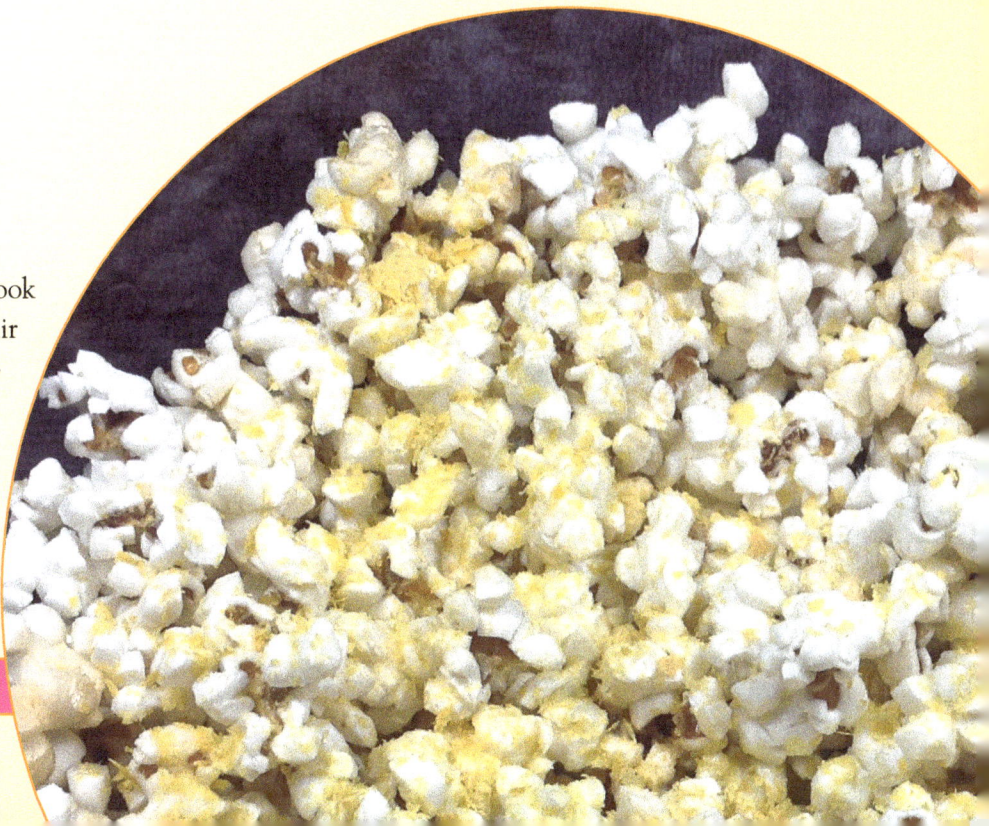

CHAPTER 5

WHAT DOES YOUR BODY DO WITH EXCESS BLOOD SUGARS?

KALE CHIPS

1 bunch of Kale

2 tbsp Apple Cider Vinegar

1 large Fresh Lemon, juiced

Nutritional Yeast

De-stem the kale. Combine the vinegar and lemon juice in a bowl. Dip the kale leaves in vinegar and lemon juice mixture and spread on a cookie sheet. Sprinkle with nutritional yeast and bake at 200 degrees until leaves are desired crispiness.

HOMEMADE TORTILLA CHIPS

Corn Tortillas

Coconut Oil

Sea Salt

Slice the corn tortillas like a pizza, into triangles. Place in a skillet with lots of coconut oil, simmer on a low heat until the triangles start to get crispy. Dash with sea salt. Allow to cool before serving.

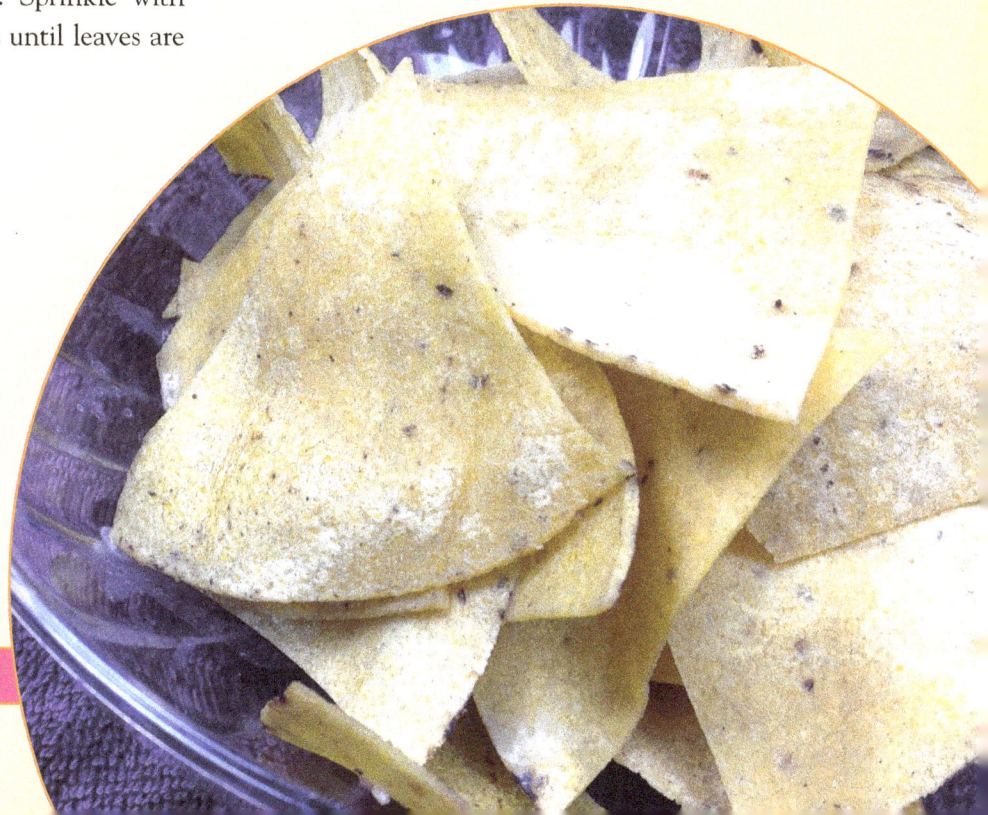

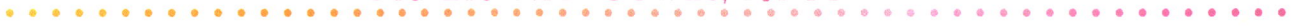

CHAPTER 5

WHAT DOES YOUR BODY DO WITH EXCESS BLOOD SUGARS?

EXCESS SUGARS ADHERE TO RED BLOOD CELLS

The process by which sugars attach to red blood cells is called "glycosylation". Glycosylation creates what is known as "hemoglobin A1c" (HgA1c), a blood marker currently used to screen for or monitor diabetes. Once glycosylation occurs, it tends to continue: as the red blood cells circulate, they combine with more glucose, thereby making more HgA1c (Pagana and Pagana 2002). According to research on HgA1c, the glycosylation process starts only after three weeks of constantly elevated sugar levels (Bunn et al. 1976) and then can be challenging to drop once it is high (Soranzo 2011).

Here is a patient lab showing elevated HgA1c:

Hemoglobin A1c

Observations	Result	Reference / UoM	Date/Status
Hemoglobin A1c [1]	● 5.8	4.8-5.6 % Above high normal	05/23/2015 06:53 am

Vendor note:
        Increased risk for diabetes: 5.7 - 6.4
        Diabetes: >6.4
        Glycemic control for adults with diabetes: <7.0			

Excess Sugars are Converted into a Fat

Your body may also convert the sugar into fatty acids. These build up inside the cell, a process called "intracellular fat build-up" (Johnson and Olefsky 2013 and Armada et al. 2012) or they can become triglycerides or cholesterol (which will show in blood work). Here is a patient lab showing high cholesterol and HgA1c:

Lipid Panel

Observations	Result	Reference / UoM	Date/Status
Cholesterol, Total [1]	● 232	100-199 mg/dL Above high normal	07/16/2015 05:10 am
Triglycerides [1]	84	0-149 mg/dL	07/16/2015 05:10 am
HDL Cholesterol [1]	75	>39 mg/dL	07/16/2015 05:13 am
Vendor note: According to ATP-III Guidelines, HDL-C >59 mg/dL is considered a negative risk factor for CHD.			
VLDL Cholesterol Cal [1]	17	5-40 mg/dL	07/16/2015 05:10 am
LDL Cholesterol Calc [1]	● 140	0-99 mg/dL Above high normal	07/16/2015 05:13 am
Comment: [1]			07/16/2015 05:13 am Not available

Hepatic Function Panel (7)

Observations	Result	Reference / UoM	Date/Status
Protein, Total, Serum [1]	7.0	6.0-8.5 g/dL	07/16/2015 04:45 am
Bilirubin, Total [1]	0.4	0.0-1.2 mg/dL	07/16/2015 04:45 am
Bilirubin, Direct [1]	0.11	0.00-0.40 mg/dL	07/16/2015 09:00 am
Alkaline Phosphatase, S [1]	115	39-117 IU/L	07/16/2015 04:49 am
AST (SGOT) [1]	21	0-40 IU/L	07/16/2015 04:49 am
ALT (SGPT) [1]	18	0-32 IU/L	07/16/2015 04:49 am

Hemoglobin A1c

Observations	Result	Reference / UoM	Date/Status
Hemoglobin A1c [1]	● 5.7	4.8-5.6 % Above high normal	07/16/2015 09:07 am

Vendor note:
    Increased risk for diabetes: 5.7 - 6.4
    Diabetes: >6.4
    Glycemic control for adults with diabetes: <7.0			

Identifying the blood sugar problem can be tricky: most patients will have normal fasting blood sugar levels, but when you test the HgA1c and look at the triglyceride or cholesterol levels, the real story can show. I always check for elevated HgA1c. Most practitioners miss it because they look at fasting glucose and only check for the HgA1c if the glucose is high. Here is an example of normal blood glucose, but high HgA1c:

Observations	Result	Reference / UoM	Date/Status
Glucose, Serum [1]	99	65-99 mg/dL	06/12/2014 06:05 am
BUN [1]	13	8-27 mg/dL	06/12/2014 06:05 am
Creatinine, Serum [1]	1.00	0.76-1.27 mg/dL	06/12/2014 06:05 am
eGFR If NonAfricn Am [1]	79	>59 mL/min/1.73	06/12/2014 06:05 am
eGFR If Africn Am [1]	91	>59 mL/min/1.73	06/12/2014 06:05 am
Hemoglobin A1c [1]	● 5.7	4.8-5.6 % Above high normal	06/12/2014 10:47 am

Vendor note:
     Increased risk for diabetes: 5.7 - 6.4
     Diabetes: >6.4
     Glycemic control for adults with diabetes: <7.0			

High/elevating blood sugars, HgA1c, and rising levels of fatty acids are hard on your immune system. Your immune system is like a street sweeper, driving through your blood vessels, tissues and organs to keep you clean of debris. High sugars, HgA1c, and excessive fatty acids clog the "streets" with debris (inflammation), making a lot of extra work for the "street sweepers".

At any given moment, you naturally have a **little bit** of inflammation in your "streets" because a **little** inflammation is used by the immune system to signal perpetual healing. It is when the inflammation is out of balance (from **over clogged** streets) that symptoms results. From work by Fitzpatric and Young (2013),

> *Inflammation is an important component of normal responses to infection and injury.* **However, chronic activation of the immune system… can lead to the establishment of a persistent inflammatory state.**

A little inflammation is a good thing, because it stimulates healing. Think of what happens when you get a cut: initially the area gets red around the cut skin. This is the immune system signaling a little inflammatory process. The little bit of inflammatory process brings the cells to the area that do the healing. But if the same area of skin continues to be cut, the cells become overwhelmed and no healing occurs, or scar tissue forms. This is likewise true with the elevated sugars, HgA1c, and fatty acid accumulation in your tissues: the inflammatory process will keep going and going as these items elevate continuously or elevate slowly over time. The inflammation of the immune system is what creates disease, as previously stated.

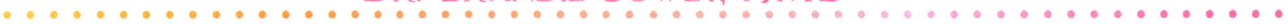

The chapters in Part Three are for those who like technical data. They highlight research connecting high blood sugars to immune system changes.

PART THREE

THE IMPACT HIGH BLOOD SUGARS HAVE ON THE IMMUNE SYSTEM

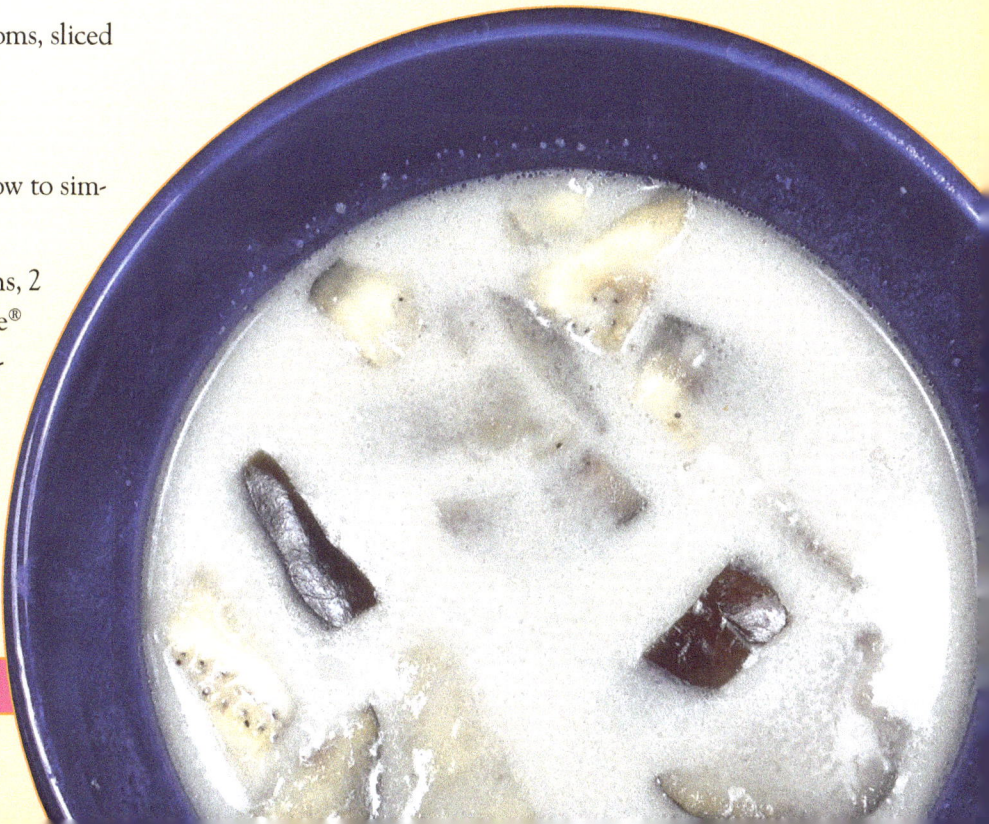

MUSHROOM SOUP

2 cups Water

1 pkg Imagine® Portobella Mushroom Soup

2 cups Beef Broth

2 Bay Leaves

1 tsp Salt

1 Onion, chopped

¼ cup Shiitake Mushrooms, chopped

1, 8 oz pkg Portobella or Shiitake Mushrooms, sliced

1 tbsp Gluten-free Tamari

1 tbsp Paprika

Add all ingredients in a cook pot and allow to simmer for 1–2 hours until flavors blend.

Variation: Add ½ cup chopped green beans, 2 additional cups Beef Broth (omit Imagine® Portobella Mushroom Soup), chopped endive or other veggies. Add a can of kidney beans in the last 15–20 minutes of cook time. This recipe also works well with ½ cup uncooked rice added in the last hour of cook time. I like to serve it with fresh sprouts on top.

CHAPTER 6

HOW HIGH BLOOD SUGARS IMPACT THE IMMUNE SYSTEM

PUM'KIN "MUFFINS"

These Pum'kin "Muffins" are free of any processed food. They do best when they are baked at a low temperature for at least an hour.

1 can Pumpkin
(or 1½ cups cooked Pie Pumpkin)

Spices (Nutmeg, Cinnamon, Cloves)

1 egg

1 can Whole Coconut Milk, fat only

Skim the fat off the liquid portion of the coconut milk. (If this is hard to do, you can freeze the can for a few hours to get the fat to separate from the watery portion of the coconut milk.)

Stir all of the ingredients together. Pour the mixture into lined muffin tins. Bake in a 350 drgree oven for about 1 hour.

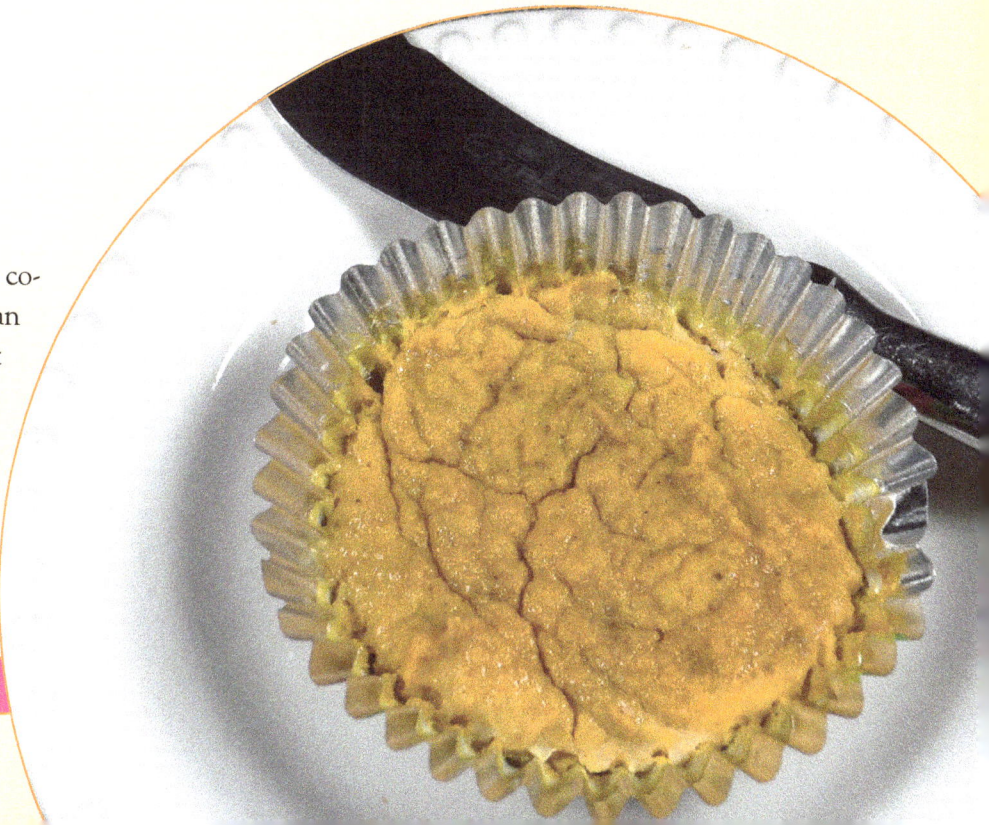

Chapter 6

How High Blood Sugars Impact the Immune System

The impact sugars have on the immune system is truly unpredictable and random, and could depend on individual genetics. Elevated or elevating blood sugars either increase or decrease cells in the immune system. These increases and decreases create chaos which we feel as symptoms or experience as disease.

Please refer to the GLOSSARY in the back of this book for the definitions of cells and medical terms discussed.

How High Blood Sugars Impact Fibroblasts

- Fibroblast activity is "altered" (Knott et al. 1999), leading to a change in the way insulin binds to cell membranes. This creates insulin resistance (Teno et al. 1999).

- Fibroblasts that normally degrade LDL's (the "bad" cholesterol") slow in activity levels (Lopes–Virella 1985), keeping LDL levels elevated.

- Fibroblasts build scar tissue. (Shamhart et al. 2014).

- Fibrinogen levels increase (Ljingman et al. 2004 and Snell–Bergeon et al. 2010) which increases inflammation.

How High Blood Sugars Impact T Cells

- Cytotoxic T cell levels increase while Helper T cells levels decrease (Richens and Jones 1985). Normally, Helper T cells keep Cytotoxic cells in check. In the presence of sugar, Helper T cells decrease too much and the Cytotoxic cells become overactive.

- Subsets of T cells called Th17 and Th1 increase in numbers and activity levels (Bogdan et al. 2011).

How High Blood Sugars Impact White Blood Cells

- White blood cell levels increase (Issan et al. 2013).

- Levels of cell signalers such as IL-1B, IL-I7, Th17, IL-6, and THF-alpha increase (Martinez et al. 2014 and Mirza et al. 2012).

- C–reactive protein (CRP) increases (Martinez et al. 2004, Mirza et al. 2012, Newton et al. 2011, and Liu et al. 2012).

- Endothelial progenitor cells levels decrease (Yue et al. 2011 and Hoffman et al. 2013).

- Vascular endothelial growth factor increases (Ozturk et al. 2009).

- White blood cells adhere to blood vessel walls, decreasing the ability of blood and nutrients to move in and out of blood vessels (Joussen et al. 2004).

- Langerhans cell density increases (Strom et al. 2014).

- White blood cell activity and response time decreases (Varga et al. 2011, Kaplar et al. 2001, Chalmers et al. 2000, Karchan et al. 2001).

- Monocytes display "abnormal" activity levels (Devaraj et al. 2011).

- Neutrophil activity changes and becomes "abnormal" (Sudo et al. 2007 and Okano et al. 2008).

- IgA, IgG, and IgM levels increase (Awartani 2010).

- Macrophage foam cell formation is enhanced (Cui et al. 2010 and Motojima et al. 2008).

- White blood cells adhere to blood vessel linings (Morigi et al. 1998).

- Natural killer cell levels decrease (Oikawa et al. 2003).

- Antibody response time to pathogens is reduced (Bhattacharya et al. 2007).

- Phagocytosis decreases (Iavicoli et al. 1982 and Marhoffer et al. 1992).

How High Blood Sugars Impact Insulin & Fat Metabolism

- Insulin resistance is driven by the build-up of fatty acids inside cells (Johnson and Olefsky 2013).

- Transcription nuclear factor KB and NF-KB (Kiechl et al. 2013) increase:

> Hepatic insulin resistance is a driving force in the pathogenesis of type 2 diabetes mellitus and is tightly coupled with excessive storage of fat and the ensuing inflammation within the liver. There is compelling evidence that activation of the transcription factor nuclear factor-kB (NF-KB) and downstream inflammatory signaling pathways systemically and in the liver are key events in the etiology of hepatic insulin resistance and B-cell dysfunction.

- Adipose tissue releases fatty acids, increasing signaling of immune system cells (Soumaya 2012), which creates inflammation.

❧ LDL levels increase.

❧ LDLs increase cortisol (Saha et al. 2013).

❧ Cholesterol transport to and from cells decreases (Zhou et al. 2008).

How High Blood Sugars Impact the Inner Workings of Cells & Antioxidant Status

❧ Mitochondria are damaged (Park et al. 2013 and van de Weijer et al. 2013).

❧ Glutathione levels decrease, contributing to oxidative damage (Waggiallah and Alzohairy 2011).

❧ DNA sustains damage (Pereira et al. 2013 and Gutman et al. 2013).

❧ mRNA function is altered, which regulates gene expression in normal physiologic functions (Corral–Fernandez et al. 2013).

❧ Oxidative stress increases (Jain et al. 2007 and Wright et al. 2006). From the researchers:

> Worldwide, there were approximately 194 million adults aged 20–79 years with diagnosed diabetes mellitus in 2003, with type 2 diabetes accounting for 90–95% of all diagnosed cases, and that number is expected to increase to 333 million over the next 20 years… a currently favored hypothesis is that the oxidative stress… is the common pathogenic factor leading to insulin resistance… and ultimately diabetes. Recently, it has been suggested that fluctuating blood glucose concentrations… may contribute significantly to oxidative stress…

❧ Telomere length decreases in skeletal muscle cells (Ahmad et al. 2012).

How High Blood Sugars Impact Clotting Pathways

❧ Factor VI levels are altered in high sugar levels (El–Ghoroury et al. 2008).

How High Blood Sugars Impact Cell Membranes

❧ Fluidity of cell membranes decreases (Bakan et al. 2006).

How High Blood Sugars Impact Cortisol Levels

❧ Cortisol levels elevate in high sugars (Godoy–Matos et al. 2006, Reynolds et al. 2010, and Mosbah et al. 2011).

SUMMARY

Changes to the immune system from chronically elevated or elevating blood sugars include:

- ❧ Lowering of antioxidants

- ❧ Increased tissue damage and inability to heal without scar tissue formation

- ❧ Changes to white blood cell function

- ❧ Damage to mitochondria of cells

- ❧ Damage to cell DNA

- ❧ Increased activity of signalers within the immune system

- ❧ Increased activity of inflammatory immune cells and cell signalers

- ❧ Increased damage to blood vessel lining

- ❧ Alteration of Cholesterol metabolism

- ❧ Increased formation of triglycerides

- ❧ Increased storage of fatty acids which then flare inflammation

VEGGIES AND RICE

1–2 cups Rice

2–3 cups Vegetables (your choice: broccoli, bok choy, onions, kale, or chard are nice), chopped

1–2 cans Coconut Milk

2 tbsp Curry Powder

Gluten-free Tamari

Salt and Pepper to taste

Cook the rice in a separate pan. While the rice is cooking, simmer the vegetables in a small amount of water. Once your veggies are cooked through, add the coconut milk, curry, tamari, and salt and pepper. Add the rice just before you are ready to serve. Heat your dish until it is warm throughout and enjoy!

DUTCH OVEN MEAL

1½ cups Water

¼ cup Rice, uncooked

¼–½ pounds Ground Buffalo or Beef, fully cooked

2 cups Vegetables (your choice), chopped

Add all ingredients to your dutch oven and allow simmer on the low for several hours, until the veggies and rice are cooked through.

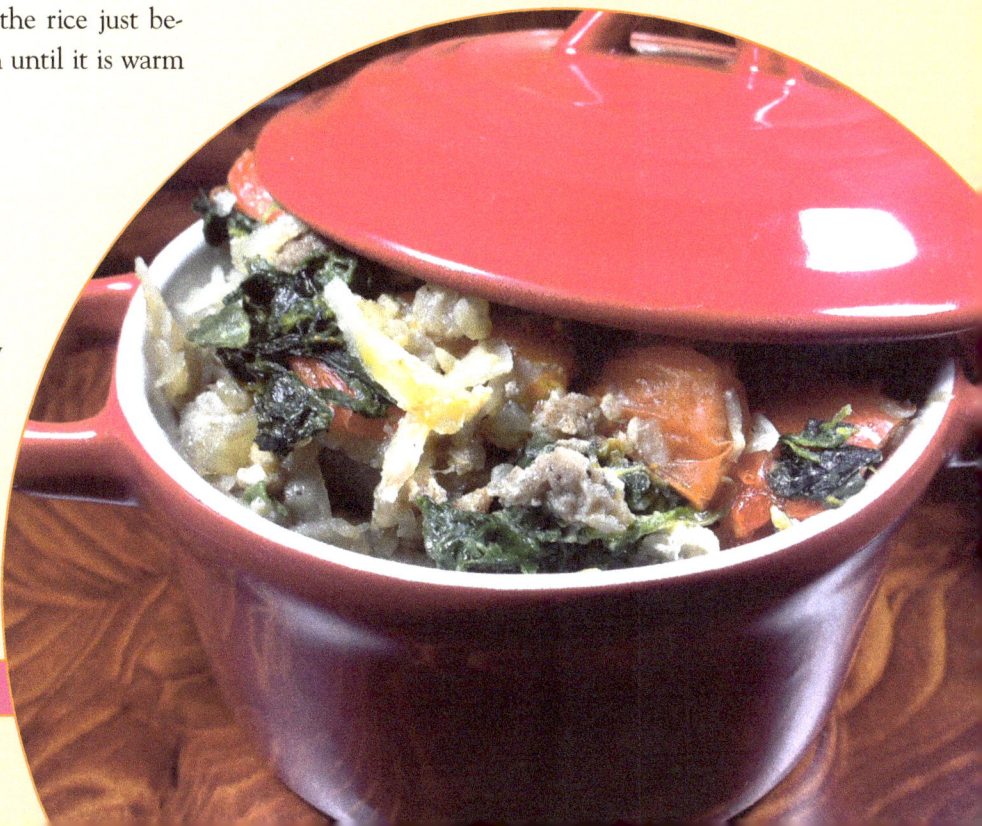

CHAPTER 7

HIGH BLOOD SUGARS & THE ROLE OF PROTEIN

CHAPTER 7

HIGH BLOOD SUGARS & THE ROLE OF PROTEIN

**High blood sugars in your body start the disease process.
Then you feed it more… with protein.**

Protein feeds inflammation, because the immune cells (which create inflammation) are built on protein.

We are taught to "detox" our bodies by consuming protein. Unfortunately, this way of thinking actually feeds the inflammation. If you try to "detox" with protein, you can and will essentially be building the inflammation. Look at this email posting that came from my medical school:

> *Make a conscious decision to give your body's main detoxification system the support and rest it needs to maintain or improve your current health picture! The 21-Day Cleanse is only $199, and includes a 3-week supply of all-natural protein drinks, a protein drink shaker, expert guidance for the cleanse process, and two group meetings and discussions. —SCNM alumna Dr. Christina Youngren*

If you want to "detox", you have to start with lowering your protein and processed sugars intake. Some protein is still good, and those who have a more athletic lifestyle will require more protein than those who are not as active. However, weight—like disease—is inflammation. When you pull processed sugars out of your diet (and moderate your protein levels), you can start to give your immune system a chance to heal.

PART FOUR

THE RELATIONSHIP BETWEEN ELEVATED BLOOD SUGARS & DISEASE

CHICKEN NUGGETS

1 Egg

2 tbsp Nutritional Yeast

2 tbsp Cornmeal (ground)

Chicken Breast, cubed

Whip the egg in a glass bowl. Combine the yeast and cornmeal in another bowl. Dip the chicken cubes in the egg, and then the yeast/cornmeal combo. Layer in a glass baking dish. Bake at 350 degrees until cooked through.

BUNLESS BURGER

Ground Beef (hormone-free, grass raised/fed)

Condiments

Large Lettuce Leaves (i.e. Butter Lettuce)

Cook your beef patty to desired "doneness". To use lettuce in place of the bun, place your patty on a bed of large lettuce leaves. Add condiments, onion, tomato or any other veggie you like. Wrap the leaves around everything. Add more leaves as needed to complete your lettuce "bun".

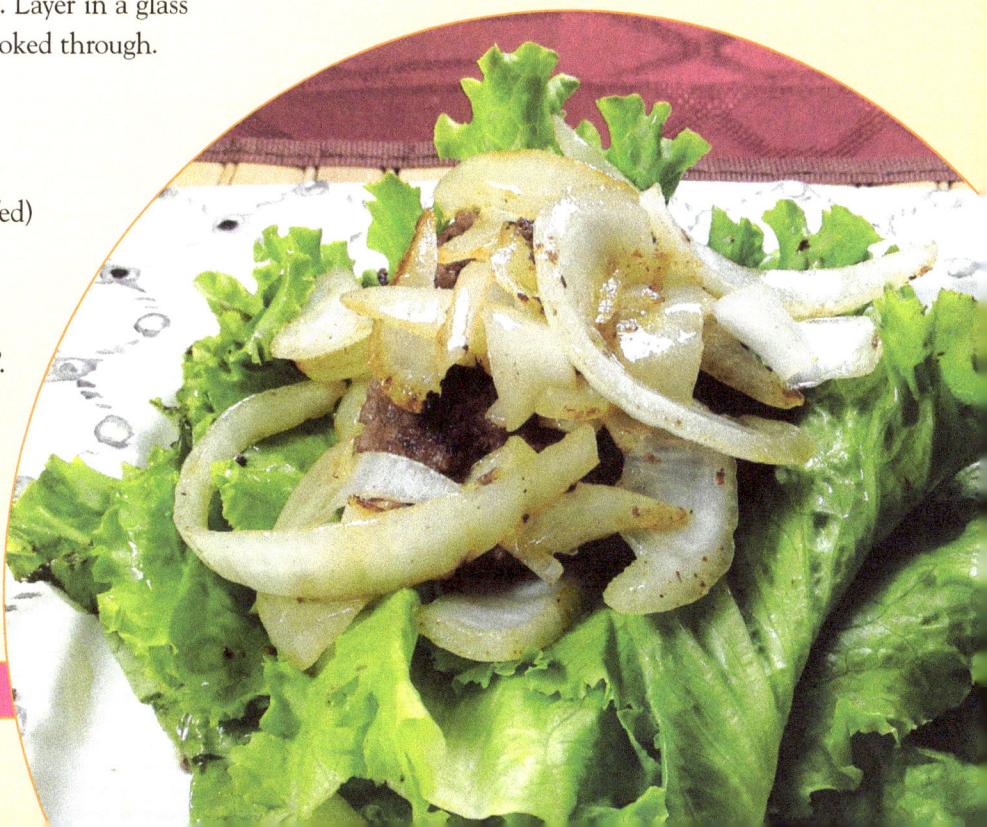

LASAGNA

1 lb Italian Sausage

1, 14.5 oz can Italian Herb Diced Tomatoes

1, 24 oz jar Newman's Own® Italian Sausage & Peppers Pasta Sauce

12 oz Extra Firm Tofu, diced

1 Onion, chopped

1 tbsp Garlic, minced (optional)

1 pkg Frozen Spinach (unthawed)

Gluten-free Lasagna Noodles (optional. Pre-cook by pkg directions)

Cook the sausage thoroughly in a saucepan. Add the tomatoes and Newman's Own® sauce. Simmer for 30–45 minutes on low. Add the onions and garlic. Simmer 5 minutes longer.

In a separate pan, sauté the tofu in butter until it starts to brown. Add the spinach and sauté for 5–10 minutes until the spinach starts to cook through.

In a 9–inch baking dish, alternately layer the meat and tomato sauce with the tofu and spinach mixture and optional gluten-free noodles. Bake, uncovered, at 350 degrees for about an hour, or until an inserted fork comes out clean.

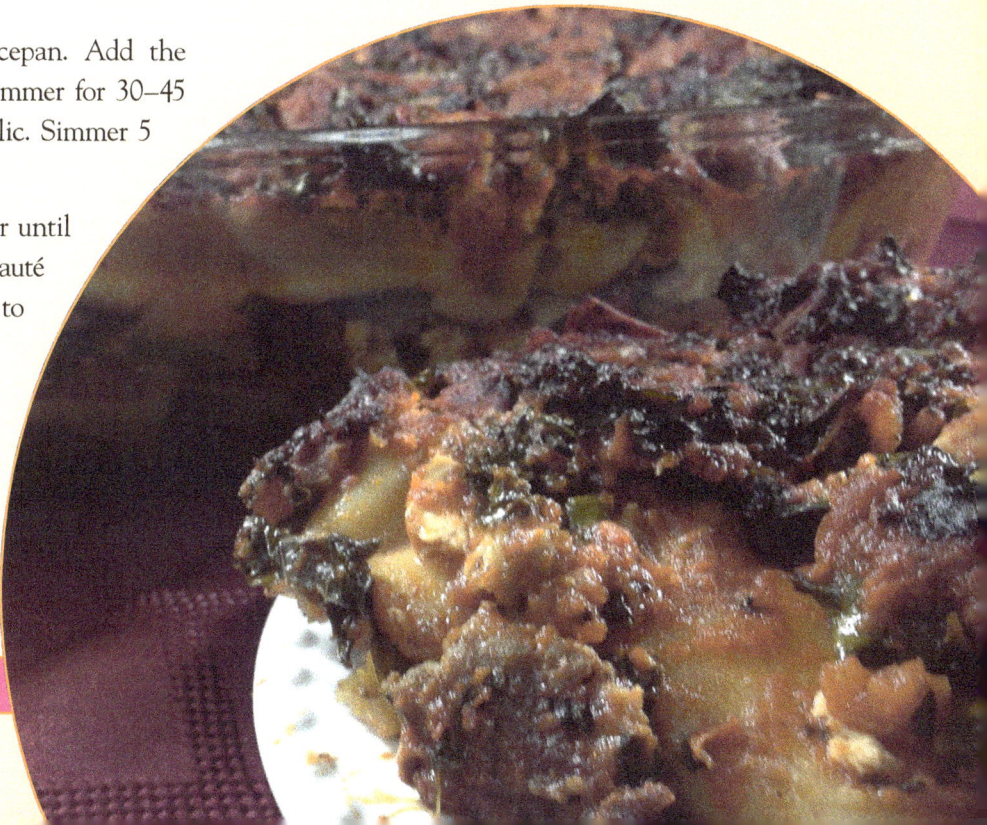

CHAPTER 8

THE RELATIONSHIP BETWEEN ELEVATED BLOOD SUGARS & CANCER

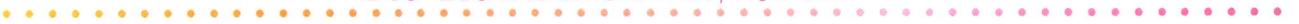

Chapter 8

The Relationship Between Elevated Blood Sugars & Cancer

The majority of cancer research is focused on genetic changes within the cell, because the prevailing theory in medicine is that genes turn on cancer. From my perspective however, our bodies were not designed to fail, they were designed to heal; therefore, I know something must trigger the genetic changes. In other words, the genes are downstream from a problem upstream. I see that one of the problems upstream is the elevated blood sugar, and that is something we can change or prevent.

It is documented in the scientific literature that **DNA changes occur in the presence of high sugars** (Czajka et al. 2015). From Stattin et al. (2007), and Coussens and Werb (2002):

> *Total cancer risk in women increased with rising plasma levels of fasting and post blood glucose… allowing for the conclusion that… hyperglycemia with total cancer risk in women and in women and men combine for several cancer sites, independently of obesity, provides further evidence for an association between abnormal glucose metabolism and cancer…*

Here is more on what research says about blood sugar levels (HgA1c) and cancer:

- Natural killer cell activity is altered and associated with HgA1c and colon cancer (Piatkiewicz et al. 2013).

- Renal cell carcinoma is associated with a high HgA1c (Habib et al. 2012).

- Caloric starvation of cancer cells decreases inflammation, shrinking tumors (Seyfried 2013).

- Fasting increases efficacy of existing cancer treatments (Safdie et al. 2012).

- High insulin levels contribute to breast and pancreatic colon cancer (Gunter et al. 2009, Onitilo et al. 2014 and Krechler et al. 2009).

- Metabolic syndrome and impaired normal glucose uptake increases colon cancer (Ashbeck et al. 2009). HgA1c is "strongly and individually associated with colorectal neoplasia" (Hsu et al. 2012).

- High sugars are associated with poor prognosis after breast cancer treatment (Krone and Ely 2005).

- Metformin use is associated with decreased risk of cancer of the colon and pancreas (Currie et al. 2009).

- Chronic hyperglycemia is "statistically significantly associated with decreased survival in survivors of early stage breast cancer " (Erickson et al. 2011).

- High fructose in the blood is associated with colorectal adenoma (Misciagna et al. 2004).

- Chemotherapy and radiation therapies may induce glucose metabolism changes (Mohn et al. 2004, Feng et al. 2013, and Mayson et al. 2013).

- Pancreatic adenocarcinoma is linked to metabolic syndrome (Wu et al. 2012).

- Obesity and insulin resistance promote endometrial cancer risk (Friedenreich et al. 2012).

- Liver damage exacerbates insulin resistance and therefore increases risk of diabetes (Duarczynski et al. 2013).

- Elevated HgA1c at time of diagnosis is linked to higher stage of cancer diagnosis (Stevens et al. 2012).

- Glucose metabolism disorders are associated with thyroid cancer (Duran et al. 2013).

- In a survey of patients at a hospital in Malaya, 32.35% of cancer patients have diabetes (Sanchez et al. 2012). "Diabetes is associated with many forms of cancer" (Dankner et al. 2012).

- Glucose metabolism issues increase the risk of childhood lymphoblastic leukemia (Skoczen et al. 2011).

- Diabetes and fasting sugar elevation is associated with non-small cell lung cancer (Luo et al. 2012 and Ortiz et al. 2012) as well as general lung cancers (Osaki et al. 2012 and Zhou et al. 2010).

- Prostate enlargement is linked to high sugars and insulin resistance (Kim et al. 2011, De Nunzio et al. 2011, Albanes et al. 2009, Bhindi et al. 2014, and Pandeye et al. 2014).

- High sugars increase breast cancer risk (Sieri et al. 2012).

- HER2 is associated with hyperglycemia (Memon et al. 2014).

- High sugars are associated with cancers of the digestive system (Mathews et al. 2010).

- Elevated serum insulin is associated with postmenopausal breast cancer (Kabat et al. 2009 and Pfeiler et al. 2009).

- Elevated serum concentration of insulin and glucose increase risk of recurrent colorectal adenomas (Flood et al. 2007).

- Ca 19-9, a tumor marker, is increased in high sugar levels (Uygar–Bayramicili et al. 2007).

SALADS

I love to make fresh salads with ingredients such as Yummy Beets. You can add any fresh veggie or fruit you desire. If you are not allergic to goat dairy, top off your greens with a little goat feta. I like to serve my salads with the oil-free dressings found at Whole Foods Market. They make a ginger-carrot oil-free dressing with their private label that is absolutely amazing.

QUINOA SALAD

1 cup Quinoa, cooked in water or Homemade Veggie Broth

½ cup Mandarin Oranges

1 cup Red Cabbage, chopped

1 cup Strawberries, diced

3-4 diced Radishes

½ cup Kale, shredded

Gluten-free Tamari

Cook the quinoa according to package directions and let cool. Add your sliced fruits and veggies and a splash of gluten-free Tamari to taste.

Variation: Add sliced cooked Chicken, a splash of Lemon Juice, Pine Nuts, or dried Cranberries.

CHAPTER 9

THE RELATIONSHIP BETWEEN ELEVATED BLOOD SUGARS & CARDIOVASCULAR DISEASE

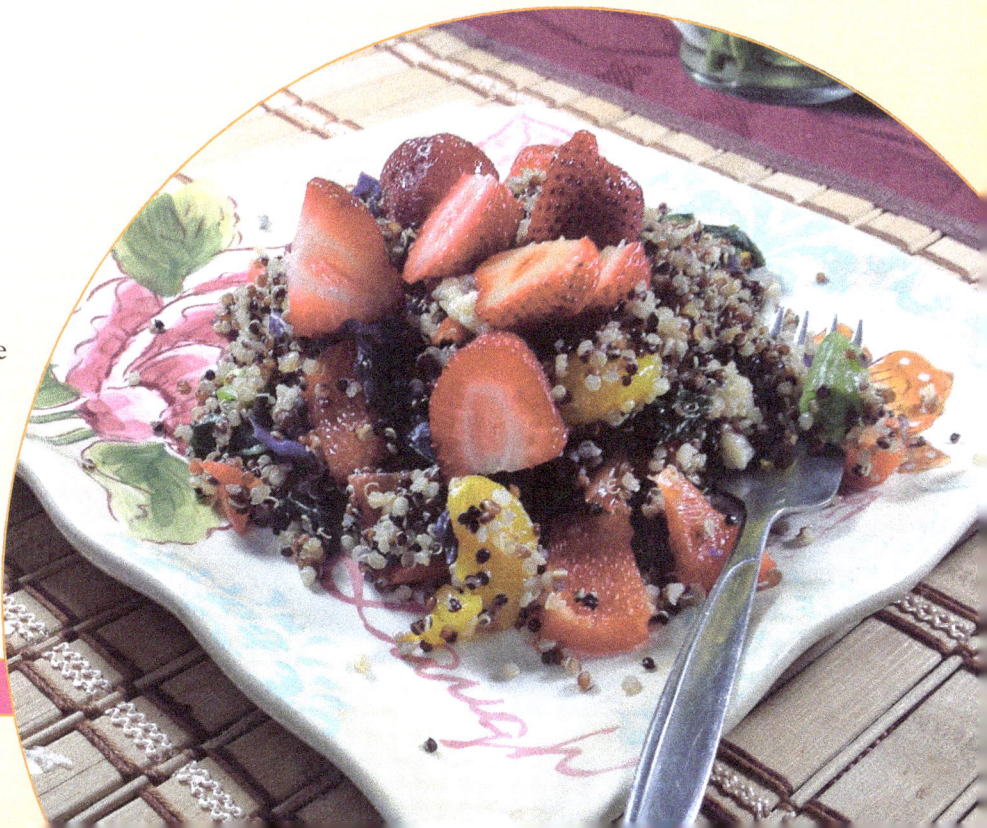

CHAPTER 9

THE RELATIONSHIP BETWEEN ELEVATED SUGARS & CARDIOVASCULAR DISEASE

A one percent rise in HgA1c is associated with a 40% increase in cardiovascular disease mortality: sugary beverage consumption on a daily basis increases cardiovascular risk exponentially (Lazzeri et al. 2014, Selvin et al. 2010, Cederberg et al. 2010, and Busko 2014).

Most of the research on sugars and cardiovascular disease relate to problems with blood vessels and especially blood vessel linings. Here are examples from the literature:

- HgA1c is associated with retinopathy, which is blood vessel damage in the eye (Massin et al. 2011).

- HgA1c contributes to stiffness of blood vessels in the heart muscle (Zieman et al. 2012).

- Sugars contribute to erectile dysfunction (Sasaki et al. 2005).

- HgA1c contributes to elevated cholesterol levels (Nishimura et al. 2011).

- Blood sugars are associated with risk of developing atrial fibrillation and stroke (Dublin et al. 2010 and Singh et al. 2013).

In other words, high sugars are actually a cause of atherosclerosis and high cholesterol (Lee and Heur 2013 and Everett et al. 2004).

In order to properly address high cholesterol, patients need to be put on protocols to impact sugar levels (Mete et al. 2011) just as much as they do elevated LDL levels. Currently, the focus is medications or supplements that only impact cholesterol.

HOMEMADE VEGGIE BROTH

You can make a very basic homemade vegetable broth with a few simple ingredients. This broth can be made in large quantities and then used to make soups or cook rice.

8 cups Water

2–3 large Onions

1 pound Carrots

1 package Celery

Salt and Pepper to taste

Chop your veggies and place in a cook pot with water. Simmer on low for 1½-2 hours. Allow the broth to cool and then strain off all the veggies. Use your broth right away, or freeze for later use. I compost the cooked veggies for my garden.

ROASTED NUTS

1 cup Raw Nuts of choice
(I like to roast macadamia nuts!)

Coconut Oil

Melt a small amount of oil in the bottom of a skillet. Add nuts. Roast for 5-10 minutes on low until the nuts begin to brown. Serve!

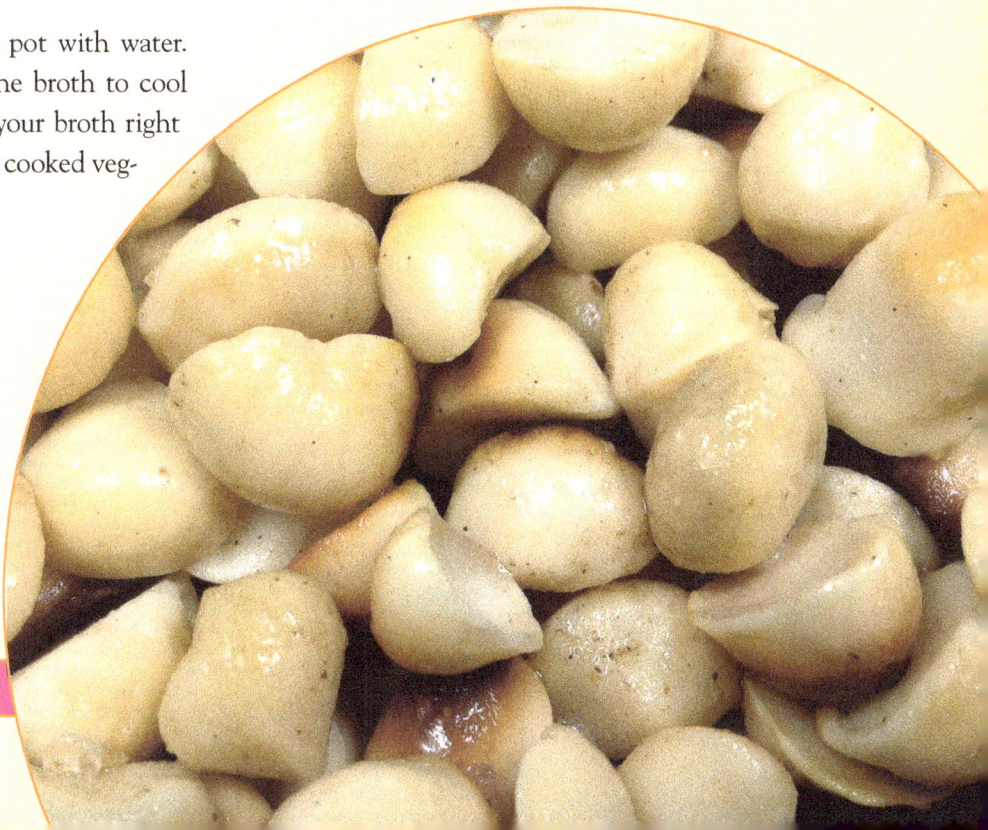

CHAPTER 10

THE RELATIONSHIP BETWEEN ELEVATED BLOOD SUGARS & INSOMNIA

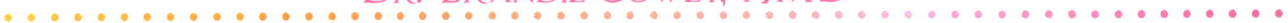

CHAPTER 10

THE RELATIONSHIP BETWEEN ELEVATED BLOOD SUGARS & INSOMNIA

Insomnia is a very common condition: many struggle to fall to sleep, while others toss and turn all night or at particular times of night. Most will wake between the hours of 1 and 3 a.m. every night.

According to Chinese medical philosophy (i.e. acupuncture philosophy), each organ has a time of day it is most active energetically. Below is a list of the major organs of the body, and the time of day they are most active:

- Lung 3–5 a.m.

- Large intestine 5–7 a.m.

- Stomach 7–9 a.m.

- Spleen 9–11 a.m.

- Heart 11 a.m.–1 p.m.

- Small intestine 1–3 p.m.

- Urinary bladder 3–5 p.m.

- Kidney 5–7 p.m.

- Pericardium (the energetic protector of the heart) 7–9 p.m.

- San jiao (the energy connecting the abdominal organs) 11 p.m.–1 a.m.

- Liver 1–3 a.m.

Notice that the liver is most active from 1–3 a.m. When the liver is out of balance, as can happen when blood sugars are high, you will wake up. The adrenals normally send a signal via the hormone cortisol to the liver, which keeps blood sugars even. But if your cortisol is high (and that can happen at night), then the signal goes to the liver at night, and you will wake up.

Changes to blood sugar regulation via the liver changes the immune system. This change is inflammatory. The inflammation keeps people up at night. Most drugs and sleep aids miss this point, and focus more on creating a sense of relaxation rather than go to this root cause. Here is some of the research agreeing with my point of view, that blood sugars control sleep:

- Diabetes is associated with shortened sleep duration, of six hours or less (Gottlieb et al. 2005, Vgontzas et al. 2009, Pyykkonen et al. 2014, and Engeda et al. 2013).

- Patients with short sleep duration secrete less insulin (Vasisht et al. 2013).

- Hyperglycemia after burn injuries creates sleep deprivation (Mayson et al. 2013).

- HgA1c and elevated blood sugars are "significantly high" in patients with short sleep duration (Nakajima et al. 2008).

- Sleep apnea is associated with high HgA1c levels (Priou et al. 2012).

- Insomnia is associated with high cortisol (Vgontzas et al. 2001) at night and too low of cortisol in the morning (Backhaus et al. 2004, Teran–Perez et al. 2012, Balbo et al. 2010, Garde et al. 2011, and Rodenbeck et al. 2002).

- IL-6 (which elevates with high sugars) and general inflammatory markers are increased in insomnia (Vgontzas et al. 2005 and Jain et al. 2012).

If you are not sleeping well, a good place to start is with a thorough investigation of your "sleep hygiene" (Udell 2005), which from my perspective means changing habits like eating that ice cream before you go to bed.

CHAPTER 11

THE RELATIONSHIP BETWEEN ELEVATED BLOOD SUGARS & MOOD

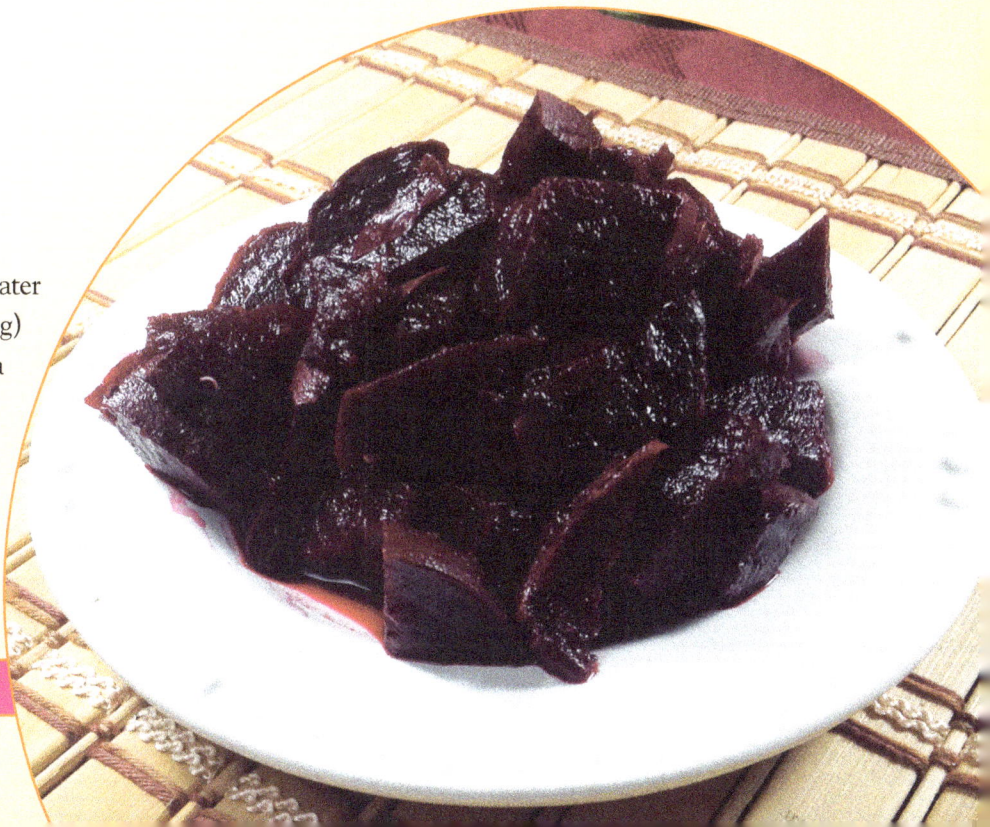

BAKED CARROTS

Carrots, sliced

Water

Butter

Stevia®

Place carrots in an oven-proof glass baking dish with a small amount of water in the bottom (to prevent the carrots from getting dehydrated). Bake in a 350 degree oven until carrots are fork-tender. Before serving, add a tbsp of melted Butter for every cup of carrots and a pinch of Stevia® to taste. This recipe is a good alternative to carrots baked in brown sugar.

YUMMY BEETS

Whole Beets, cleaned and trimmed

White Vinegar

Water

Put the whole beets and a small amount of water (to prevent dehydration during cooking) in a glass baking dish. Bake, covered, in a 250 degree oven until a fork tender. Place the beets in a glass jar. Cover completely with vinegar. Leave overnight in the refrigerator. Remove in the morning and serve as desired. A truly yummy treat! You can re-use the vinegar a few times.

Chapter 11

The Relationship Between Elevated Blood Sugars & Mood

Just as with insomnia, the research connecting elevated blood sugar and depression/anxiety is staggering. Here are a few of the studies that summarize a 3000 plus literature review I conducted while writing this book:

- Major depressive disorder is associated with diabetes (Mezuk et al. 2013 and Katon 2010), and can be two times higher in diabetic patients than in non-diabetic patients (Siddiqui et al. 2014).

- Depressive symptoms increase risk of insulin resistance (Khambaty et al. 2014).

- Depression, Alzheimer's, and impaired glucose metabolism are linked (Marano et al. 2014).

- Metformin creates anti-depressant effects by treating the high sugars (Guo et al. 2014).

- IL-6 (a cell signaler) tends to be elevated in patients with depression (Rudolf et al. 2014).

CHAPTER 12

THE RELATIONSHIP BETWEEN ELEVATED BLOOD SUGARS, ARTHRITIS & NERVOUS SYSTEM CONDITIONS

HOMEMADE COCONUT MILK

¼ cup Unsweetened Coconut Shavings

2 cups Boiling Water

Pour coconut shavings into a blender and cover with the boiling water. Allow to steep for 5 minutes; then cover and blend. Strain and reserve the coconut shavings and resultant liquid milk. Use the reserved shavings to make 1 or 2 more batches of milk. Compost or discard the used shavings. Serve with spices, if desired.

HOMEMADE CHAI

Unsweetened Milk of choice (I like to use Almond Milk)

1 bag, Black Tea

Cinnamon and Nutmeg

Heat milk to desired temperature, pour into cup, add the black tea bag, and sprinkle with spices. Allow to steep before drinking.

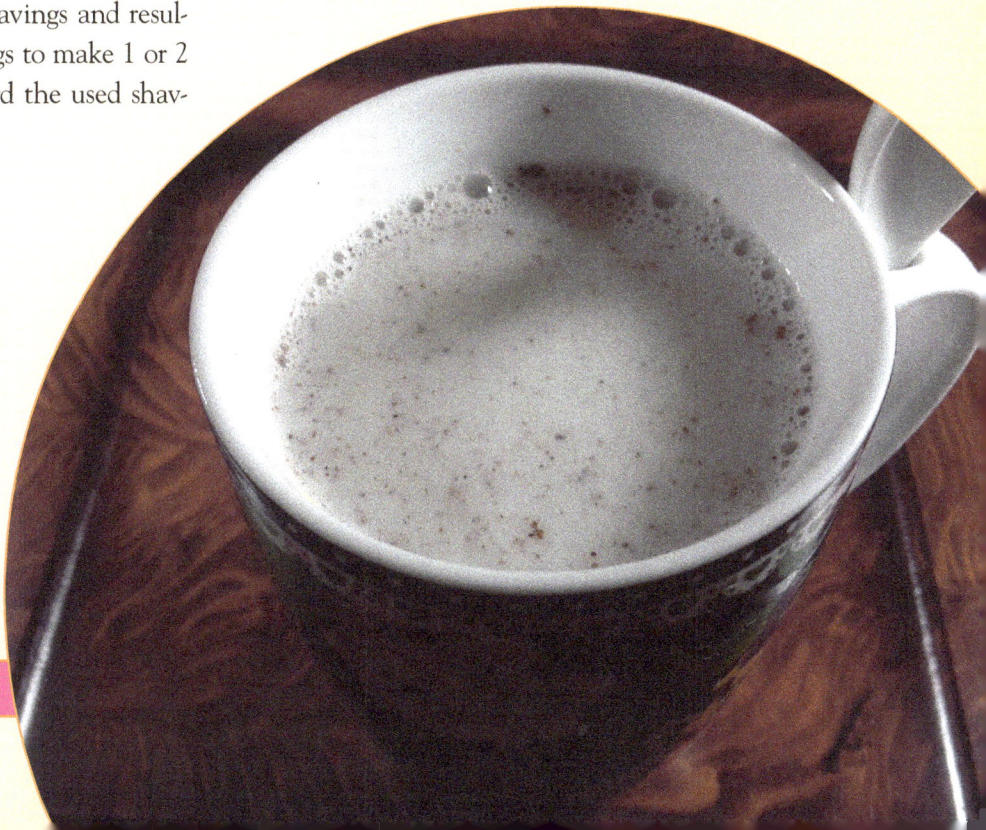

Chapter 12

The Relationship Between Elevated Blood Sugars, Arthritis & Nervous System Conditions

Orthopedic conditions are worsened by—and can be created by—elevated blood sugars (Lebiedz–Odrobina and Kay 2010). Below are some of the highlights of an extensive literature review. Most of the research is focused on changes in immune cell signaler activity (due to the elevated blood sugars), which leads to the nervous system or orthopedic condition.

- IL-17, IL-1, IL-6, IL-1B, IL-22, IL-10, TNF alpha, and CD8 T cells are flared by high blood sugars which flare rheumatoid arthritis (Matuszewska 2014, Hussein et al. 2008, Magyari et al. 2014, and Leipe et al 2014).

- High blood sugars increase IL-23 and IL-17, which are involved in spondyloarthritic development (Smith and Colbert 2014).

- HgA1c creates over-activity or activation of IL-17, which then creates autoimmune arthritis of joints and decreases collagen in the joint space (Corneth et al. 2014).

- Sugars increase IL-6 which is active in the synovial fluid of arthritic joints (Honke et al. 2014 and Wada et al. 2014).

- IL-8 (increased by blood sugars) is involved in joint inflammation (Valcamonica et al. 2014).

- High blood sugars promote abnormal B cell response and later activate IL-6, contributing to polyarthralgia rheumatism (van der Geest et al. 2014).

- Sugars promote IL-17 which activates fibroblasts, and when over-active, contribute to joint diseases and scar tissue development (Lee et al. 2014).

- Abnormal expression of CD4 and CD8 T cells turn on IL-21. This increases autoimmune inflammation (Iwamoto et al. 2014).

- Sugars suppress B cells that normally regulate the over-activity of the immune system (Daien et al. 2014).

- Blood sugars increase IL-6 and IL-1B secretion, which then increase cartilage degradation (Yang et al. 2014, Lenski and Scherer 2014, and Liu et al. 2104).

The cell signaler IL-6 is part of many different disease processes (Franck et al. 2014, De Filippo et al. 2014, and Allen et al. 2014), but is especially active in arthritic conditions. Look at how complicated its interactions are (pathwaycommons.org):

Because of the activity of immune particles such as IL-6, arthritic conditions are often associated with nervous system diseases. For example, a study in 2013 used imaging to watch the movement of immune cells within the blood. What was discovered is that immune cells move around more than what was previously known, and that they actually go from the bloodstream to the central nervous system playing an "unexpected role" in not only systemic diseases, but also neurological (Zenaro et al. 2013). This leads to disease processes as demonstrated by these studies:

- Demyelination in multiple sclerosis (MS) is caused by overactive T cells such as Th1 and Th17 (Trenova et al. 2014, Xiao et al. 2014, and Profumo et al. 2012). These are the T cells turned on by high blood sugar levels.

- IL-1B is associated with MS brain lesions, showing higher levels in cerebral spinal fluid (CSF) levels (Seppi et al. 2014). IL-1B is one of the most common cell signalers turned on by elevated blood sugars.

- IL-1B in the CSF is associated with progression of MS (Rossi et al. 2014).

- IL-8 is higher in CSF of MS patients (Matejcikova et al. 2014).

Autoimmune conditions such as Lupus, scleroderma, or airway diseases all come from the same root cause as do arthritic or nervous system diseases: immune cells and cell signalers flared by sugars. Here is what some of the research has to say (remembering that the "IL", or interleukins, are all turned on by high blood sugars):

- IL-133 is associated with airway diseases (Mizutuni et al. 2013).

- IL-17 is associated with emphysema (Kurimoto et al. 2013).

Abnormal T cell activity is associated with autoimmune conditions (Profano et al. 2012, Pan et al. 2013, Lyn-Cook et al. 2014, Ma et al. 2014, Jolly et al. 2014, Zhao et al. 2014, Aghdashi et al. 2013, Lan et al. 2014, and Gao et al. 2014).

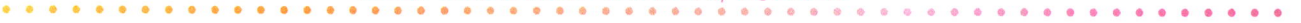

The chapters in Part Five highlight how you can live a healthier lifestyle without processed sugar.

PART FIVE

HOW TO LIVE THE SWEET LIFE

BEEF BROTH

Dr. Tallman (arizonaprolotherapy.com) would tell you homemade beef broth soup is essential for building joints and connective tissue. I would say its essential for building chi. Either way, you can't go wrong. It is easiest made in a crock pot rather than on the stove top. On the stove it tends to cook too fast and forms a fatty, foamy film on top. Made in the crock pot, you get a perfect beef broth that you can add veggies, rice, or rice noodles to, or sip on its own, with or without added salt.

1–2   Beef Soup Bones (depending on your crock pot's capacity)

Water

Fill crock pot with water and add the soup bones to it. Simmer on low setting over night. Add desired veggies.

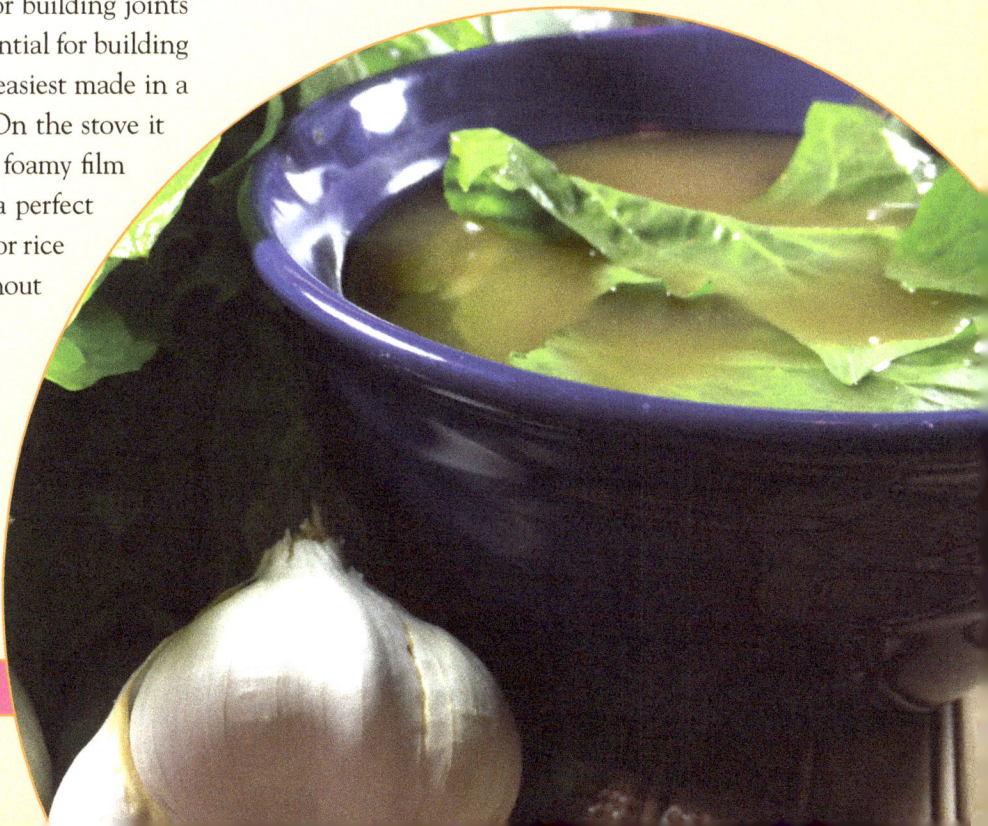

CHAPTER 13

STAYING HEALTHY

BERRY CONCENTRATE

1, 10 oz pkg Mango

1, 10 oz pkg Berries of choice

Spices (i.e. Cinnamon or Nutmeg)

Salt

Place fruit in a saucepan over low heat. Stir slowly until most of the fruit liquid evaporates. Remove from heat. Cool slightly. Sprinkle with spice(s) and a pinch of salt. Serve warm or topped with Homemade Coconut Whip.

HOMEMADE COCONUT WHIP

2 cans Whole Coconut Milk (Whole Foods Market 365 label is excellent for this recipe)

Spices (Cinnamon or other spice)

The fat from coconut milk settles on the top of this product, with the liquid on the bottom. (Other coconut oils do not separate as readily.) Slim off the fat. (If this is hard to do, freeze the can for a few hours until the fat separates.) Whip the separated fat in a blender. Add a small amount of the coconut liquid if your whip is too thick. Add a pinch of spice, if desired.

Variation: Homemade Coconut Whip is excellent with ½ cup Cherry Juice added during the blending.

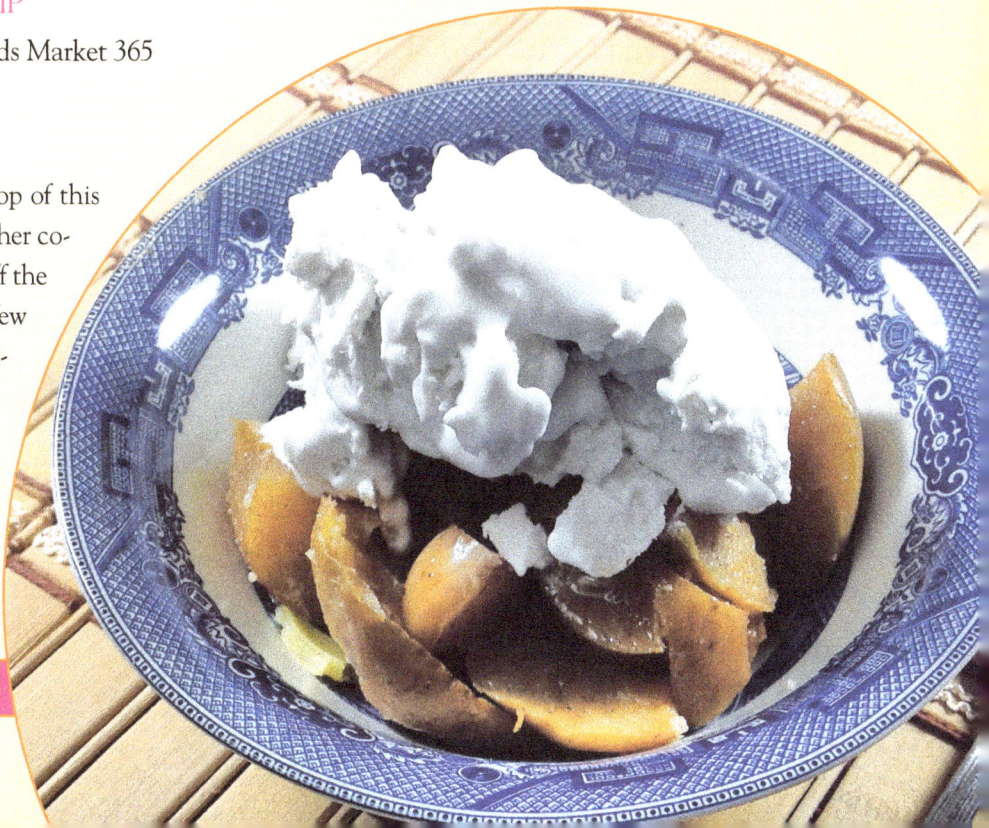

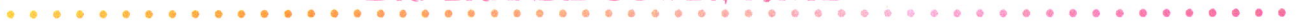

Chapter 13

Staying Healthy

The situation is not hopeless! There is so much you can do to keep the cells of your body happy and healthy. You can live without added sugars or processed foods in your diet! You can eat a simple, satisfying, color-rich diet full of minerals, vitamins, and antioxidants that has moderate protein and fat levels. Balance is key, as well as continuous avoidance of processed foods and sugars as much as possible. Here is a food pyramid I live by:

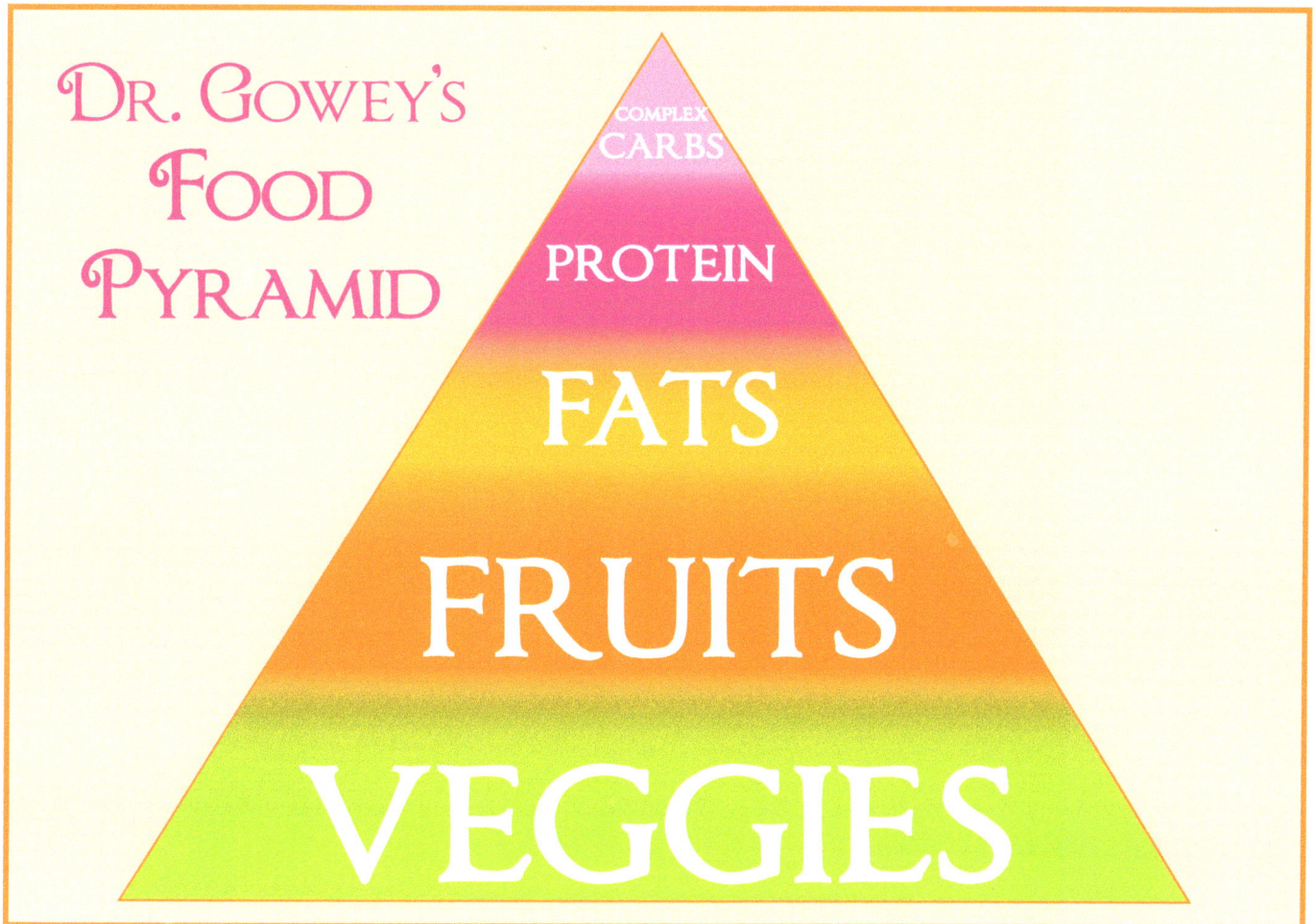

Dr. Gowey's Food Pyramid

COMPLEX CARBS
PROTEIN
FATS
FRUITS
VEGGIES

From the Research Literature, Here Are Things You Can Do

- Avoid artificial sweeteners. They are linked to glucose intolerance (Skwarecki 2014).

- Consume a diet high in antioxidants to protect against oxidative stress (Sharhan et al. 2008). Oxidative stress promotes and drives inflammation.

- Exercise to reduce inflammation (Giallaurin et al. 2008) and insulin resistance (Ligibel et al. 2008).

The key to exercise is doing something you enjoy and that which gives you either time alone or time with friends. What are some of your favorite activities? I had a diabetic patient reduce her fasting a.m. sugars from the 300s to 170 with a few weeks of daily walking. She would walk anywhere from 2–6 miles a day. Or you can throw in a little tai chi or yoga, as even these improve blood sugar levels and T-helper cell function (Yeh et al. 2009).

- Caloric restriction decreases cell signalers (i.e. IL-6), neutrophils, and CRP (Imaygama et al. 2012 and Neuhousen et al. 2012).

Fasting has long been known to decrease conditions such as diabetes and cancer.

- Keep high-fat dairy and dairy foods with added sugar out of your diet, as they are associated with breast cancer (Kroenke and Caan et al. 2013).

If you have a child with symptoms such as ear infections, chronic bronchial infections, pneumonia, or eczema, they have a food sensitivity. The most common sensitivity is dairy, and oftentimes wheat products. If you are breastfeeding, get off dairy. If your child is eating solids, get them off the dairy (and possibly gluten-containing foods) and their symptoms over several months will dissipate. There is no reason to put drain tubes in your child's ears or keep them on repeat bouts of antibiotics. Early age sensitivity to foods carries into adulthood, and contributes to more serious conditions as we age, such as diabetes.

- Keep Vitamin C levels high. Low Vitamin C levels lead to damage to cells if blood sugar levels are high (Franke et al. and Kodama et al. 1994).

Be careful how much Vitamin C you consume or get via IV therapies. I know physicians who use 100 grams or more of Vitamin C per IV, and this can actually potentiate cortisol (Kodana et al. 1994 and Padayatty et al. 2007). And as we have learned, cortisol tells the liver to release sugar stores (see page 48, Kodama et al. 1994). I always check the patient's fasting blood sugars and HgA1c prior to any administration of high dose Vitamin C IV infusions.

- Consuming meals with spices such as turmeric will help regulate the over-activity of the immune system cells, in particular IL-6 (Jain et al. 2009).

Monitoring and eliminating excessive caffeinated beverages from your diet reduces HgA1c (clinical experience).

🔸 Green tea decreases glucose levels and insulin resistance (Huang et al. 2013).

If I have a patient who over did it on alcohol, I tell them to have some nice organic green tea, as it always helps get the blood sugar back into balance.

🔸 Avoid toxic exposures as best you can. In my practice, I have seen how toxins such as pesticides, bisphenol A, phalates, dioxins, fluorinated chemicals, and heavy metals can create blood sugar problems.

While it is difficult to avoid all chemicals (since we live in a world of manufactured products) you can still do things to keep the chemicals from building up excessively in your tissues. Exercise and infrared sauna are two easy tools you can use, as the action of sweating moves toxins out of the body through the skin. You can also avoid use of plastics for storing your foods or beverages. Phalates are known compounds in plastics that contribute to the development of cancer.

🔸 Low levels of magnesium are associated with high HgA1c (Sjorgren et al. 1986).

The best magnesium I have seen is a powdered calcium and magnesium formulation made by Thorne. It absorbs well.

🔸 Keep antioxidants (these are fruits and veggies with color, such as berries or peppers) high in your diet. Low levels of antioxidants contribute to white blood cell dysfunction (Akkus et al. 1996 and Yasunari et al. 2002).

From my food pyramid on page 63, I put veggies and colorful fruits at the bottom of the food pyramid as they are known to decrease DNA damage (Mullner et al. 2013). DNA damage is what leads us to sugar problems, and diseases such as cancer!

🔸 Keep adrenal cortisol levels healthy with adrenal supportive herbs. Cortisol levels go up under stress, especially chronic stress (clinical experience).

I recommend herbs such as Maca, Rhodiola, and Withania.

🔸 Gardening lowers HgA1c activity (Weltin and Lavin 2012).

🔸 Omega oils decrease insulin resistance (Rafraf et al. 2012).

I recommend patients take 3–4 grams of Omega oils daily. My preference is fish oil.

🔸 Using medicinal herbs such as Astragalus protects the cell DNA, lowers the cell signalers, and prevents mitochondrial damage (Soromou et al. 2012, Percival et al. 2012, and Schmid et al. 2009).

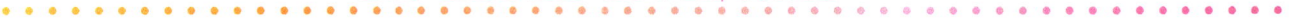

CHAPTER 14

CONCLUDING REMARKS

FROZEN BLACK CHERRIES

I like to munch on partially thawed Frozen Organic Cherries if I have any sugar cravings. They help to balance blood sugar.

BAKED APPLES

Apples, sliced (enough to fill a crock pot)

Spices (i.e. Cinnamon, Nutmeg, or Cloves)

Butter

Slice the apples into sections and place in crock pot. Add 1–2 tsp butter (depending on size of crock pot). Add any desired spices. Set at a low temperature and allow to cook slowly. Serve when apples are cooked through (fork goes in smoothly). This is wonderful topped with Homemade Coconut Whip.

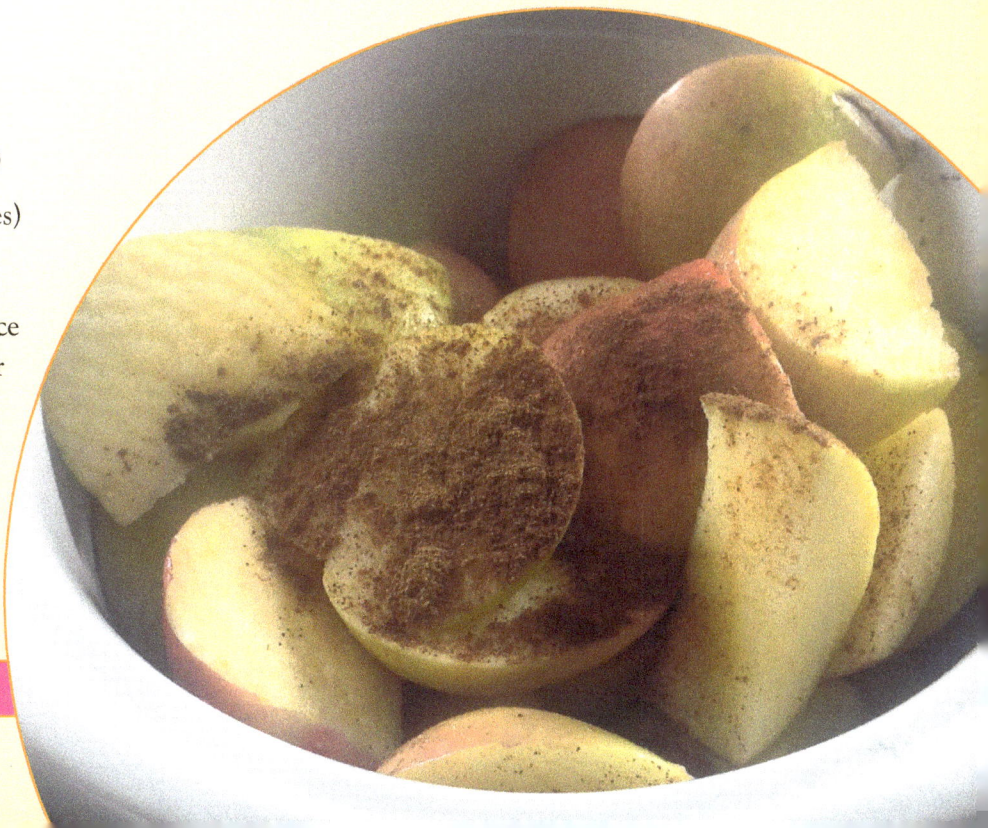

CHAPTER 14

CONCLUDING REMARKS

Patients come in my office sick, but if they keep believing and don't give up, we always figure out ways to best support them and decrease symptoms. My advice to everyone I treat is to always believe in the healing power of the body, and to not give up. Those who give up are those who never achieve healing. Never give up. You need to stay open and see how the answers come.

I think one of the main issues with the current health care system is the lack of understanding of the immune system. The immune system cells are what create inflammation. And as I have tried to show with this book, the inflammation is what creates disease, from cancer to arthritis. I encourage you to consider the information I have presented in this book, and make strides to limit your exposure to sugar, or to anything that may raise blood sugar levels.

Patients always tell me (at first) that sugar is "the hardest to change and there is no way I will I love it too much". But then we start the work of healing on so many levels and using herbs in the right ways at the right time, and they start to shift on their own. Then they come to me saying how much they can't believe they thought they needed all those processed foods and sugars. And how they are more aware of those around them "on the corporate processed food conveyor belt" (the words of Laura Brummels).

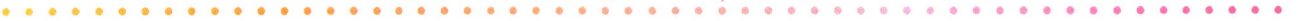

PART SIX

APPENDIX

NO-SUGAR ICE CREAM

2 cans Whole Coconut Milk (not Lite)

Spices (i.e. Cinnamon, Nutmeg, Cloves)

Pour the coconut milk into a baking dish lined with parchment paper (sonnetskitchen.com) and place in the freezer. When it's frozen, break into chunks and blend on high. You may add cinnamon or other spices before serving. You can also add a pinch of Stevia® or Cherry Juice if you so desire.

NO-SUGAR CHOCOLATE TREATS

$1/8$ tsp Stevia®

4 tbsp Cocoa Butter

4 squares Baker's Unsweetened Cocoa
(or 4 tbsp Cocoa Powder)

1 tbsp Coconut Oil

Melt all these ingredients together and pour into molds. For an even yummier treat, dip Strawberries in the chocolate mix and allow to cool on wax paper.

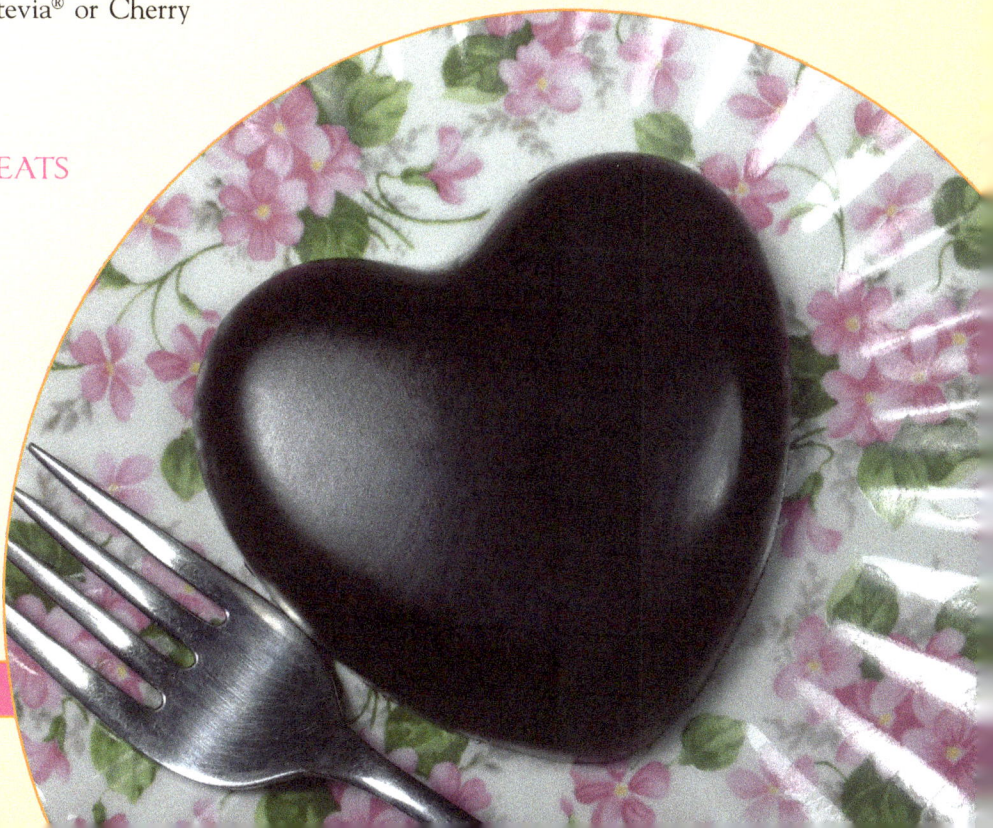

GLOSSARY

❧ **Antibody:** A type of immune cell (IgG or IgM) that has a memory for a pathogen

❧ **C-reactive protein** (CRP): An inflammatory marker that can be ordered in blood work

❧ **Cells signalers:** Proteins that tell cells what to do, they include interleukins (IL) such as IL-1B, IL-17, or IL-6

❧ **Cortisol:** Hormone made by the adrenals that regulates energy, mood, sleep/wake cycles, focus, memory, blood pressure, the immune system, and absorption of nutrients

❧ **Cytotoxic T cells:** Cells that respond to pathogens/inflammation

❧ **Endothelial progenitor cells:** Cells that build blood vessels

❧ **Factor VI:** Part of your clotting pathway

❧ **Fibrinogen:** An inflammatory marker produced by the liver

❧ **Fibroblasts:** Cells that are designed to continually heal, create and rebuild tissues and organ systems

❧ **Helper T cells:** Cells that keep tissues free of inflammation and keep the Cytotoxic T cells in check

❧ **IgA, IgA and IgM:** Types of white blood cells that build memory to pathogens, respond to food sensitivities, and play a role in maintaining the gut lining

❧ **Insulin:** A hormone that helps bring sugars into cells

❧ **Insulin resistance:** The inability of cells to respond to the presence of insulin when it brings sugar to the cell

❧ **Langerhans cells:** White blood cells in the skin that respond to pathogens such as viruses or bacteria

❧ **LDLs:** "Bad" cholesterol"

❧ **Macrophage foam cell:** A compilation of macrophage cells and immune signalers/fats

❧ **Mitochondria:** Part of the cell that creates energy

❧ **Monocytes:** A type of white blood cell

❧ **Natural killer cells:** Cells that respond to pathogens like viruses

❧ **Oxidative stress:** Low antioxidant level (which leads to tissue damage)

❧ **Phagocytosis:** The way white blood cells engulf pathogens to eliminate them

- **Scar tissue:** Over-creation of tissues, built by fibroblasts
- **Telomere:** Part of your genetic blueprint that protects chromosomes from damage
- **Th17 and Th1:** Types of Helper T cells
- **Transcription nuclear factor KB**: A protein that increases cell division
- **Vascular endothelial growth factor:** A protein that signals the building of blood vessel linings
- **White blood cells:** Cells that respond to pathogens (such as viruses or bacteria), including neutrophils, basophils, monocytes, and macrophages

References

Ahmad, S., et al. *Telomere length in blood and skeletal muscle in relation to measures of glycaemia and insulinaemia.* Diabet Med. 2012 Oct;29(10):e377-81.

Aghdashi, M., et al. *Serum levels of IL-18 in Iranian females with systemic lupus erythematosus.* Med Arch. 2013;67(4):237-40.

Akkus, I., et al. *Leukocyte lipid peroxidation, superoxide dismutase, glutathione peroxidase and serum and leukocyte vitamin C levels of patients with type II diabetes mellitus.* Clin Chim Acta. 1996 Jan 31;244(2):221-7.

arizonaprolotherapy.com

Asare, Y., et al. *The vascular biology of macrophage migration inhibitory factor (MIF). Expression and effects in inflammation, atherogenesis and angiogenesis.* Throb Haemost. 2013 Jan 17;109(3).

Ashbeck, E., et al. *Components of metabolic syndrome and metachronous colorectal neoplasia.* Cancer Epidemiol Biomarkers Prev. 2009 Apr;18(4):1134-43.

authoritynutrition.com

Awartani, F. *Serum immunoglobulin levels in type 2 diabetes patients with chronic periodontitis.* J Contemp Dent Pract. 2010 May 1;11(3):001-8.

Backhaus, J., et al. *Sleep disturbances are correlated with decreased morning awakening salivary cortisol.* Psychoneuroendocrinology. 2004 Oct;29(9):1184-91.

Bakan, E., et al. *Effects of type 2 diabetes mellitus on plasma fatty acid composition and cholesterol content of erythrocyte and leukocyte membranes.* Acta Diabetol. 2006 Dec;43(4):109-13.

Balbo, M., et al. *Impact of sleep and its disturbances on hypothalamo-pituitary-adrenal axis activity.* Int J Endocrinol. 2010; 759234.

Bhattacharya, S., et al. *Polymorphonuclear leukocyte function in type-2 diabetes mellitus patients and its correlation with glycaemic control.* Nepal Med Coll J. 2007 Jun;9(2):111-6.

Bhindi, B., et al. *Dissecting the association between metabolic syndrome and prostate cancer risk: analysis of a large clinical cohort.* Eur Urol. 2014 Feb 14.

Bogdan, J. and Madhumita, M., et al. *Elevated proinflammatory cytokine production by a skewed T cell compartement requires monocytes and promotes inflammation in Type 2 diabetes.* Jnt of Immuno. 2011 Jan;136(2): 1162-1172.

Brooks, M. *Anti-inflammatories May Help Ease Depression.* Medscape.com, 10/21/14.

Bunn, H., et al. *The biosynthesis of human hemoglobin A1c. Slow glycosylation of hemoglobin in vivo.* J Clin Invest. 1976 Jun;57(6):1652-1659.

Busko, M. *A soda a day ups CVD risk by 30%: NHANES Study.* Medscape posting. 2014 Feb 4.

Cederberg, H., et al. *Postchallenge glucose, A1C, and fasting glucose as predictors of type 2 diabetes and cardiovascular disease.* Diabetes Care. 2010 Sep;33(9):2077-83.

Chalmers, A., et al. *Lymphocyte 5 ectonucleotidase: an indicator of oxidative stress in humans?* Redox Rep. 2000;5(2-3):89-91.

Corneth, O., et al. *Absense of interleukin-17 receptor a signaling prevents autoimmune inflammation of the joint and leads to a Th2-like phenotype in collagen-induced arthritis.* Arthritis Rheumatol. 2014 Feb;66(2):340-9.

Coussens, L. and Werb, Z. *Inflammation and cancer.* Nature. 2002 Dec 19-26;420(6917):860-7.

Cui, X., et al. *Macrophage foam cell formation is augmented in serum from patients with diabetic angiopathy.* Diabetes Res Clin Pract. 2010 Jan;87(1):57-63.

Currie, C., et al. *The influence of glucose-lowering therapies on cancer risk in type 2 diabetes.* Diabetologia. 2009 Sep;52(9):1766-77.

Daien, C., et al. *Regulatory B10 cells are decreased in patients with rheumatoid arthritis and are inversely correlated with disease activity.* Arthritis Rheumatol. 2014 Aug;66(8):2037-46.

Dankner, R., et al. *Effect of elevated basal insulin on cancer incidence and mortality in cancer incident patients: the Israel GOH 29-year follow-up study.* Diabetes Care. 2012 Jul;35(7):1538-43.

De Filippo, G., et al. *IL-6, soluble IL-6 receptor /IL-6 complex and insulin resistance in obese children and adolescents.* J Endocrinol Invest. 2015 Mar;38(3):339-43.

De Nunzio C., et al. *Metabolic syndrome is associated with high grade gleason score when prostate cancer is diagnosed on biopsy.* Prostate. 2011 Feb 25.

Devaraj, S., et al. *Demonstration of increased toll-like receptor 2 and toll-like receptor 4 expression in monocytes of type 1 diabetes mellitus patients with microvascular complications.* Metabolism. 2011 Feb;60(2):256-9.

Dublin, S., et al. *Diabetes mellitus, glycemic control, and risk of atrial fibrillation.* Journal of Gen. Int. Med. 2010 Aug;25(8):853-858.

Duran, A., et al. *The relationship between glucose metabolism disorders and malignant thyroid disease.* Int J Clin

Oncol. 2013 Aug;18(4):585-9.

Durczynski, A., et al. *Major liver resection results in early exacerbation of insulin resistance, and may be a risk factor of developing overt diabetes in the future.* Surg Today. 2013 May;43(5):534-8.

El-Ghoroury, E., et al. *Study of factor Vii, tissue factor pathway inhibitor and monocyte tissue factor in noninsulin-dependent diabetes mellitus.* Blood Coagul Fibrinolysis. 2008 Jan;19(1):7-13.

Engeda, J., et al. *Association between duration and quality of sleep and the risk of pre-diabetes: evidence from NHANES.* Diabet Med. 2013 Jun;30(6):676-80.

Erickson, K., et al. *Clinically defined type 2 diabetes mellitus and prognosis in early-stage breast cancer.* J Clin Oncol. 2011 Jan 1;29(1):54-60.

Everett, B., et al. *Interleukin-18 and the risk of future cardiovascular disease among initially healthy women.* Atherosclerosis. 2004 Jan. 202(1): 282-8.

Feng J., et al. *Secondary diabetes associated with 5-fluorouracil-based chemotherapy regimens in non-diabetic patients with colorectal cancer: results from a single-centre cohort study.* Colorectal Dis. 2013 Jan;15(1):27-33.

Fitzpatrick, M. and Young, S. *Metabolomics, a novel window into finalmatory disease.* Medical Intelligence. 2013;143.

Flood, A., et al. *Elevated serum concentrations of insulin and glucose increase risk of recurrent colorectal adenomas.* Gastro. 2007 Nov;133(5):1423-9.

Franke, S., et al. *Vitamin C intake reduces the cytotoxidcity associated with hyperglycemia in prediabetes and type 2 diabetes.* Biomed Res Int'l. 2013 Article ID 896536, 6 pages.

Friedenreich, C., et al. *Case-control study of markers of insulin resistance and endometrial cancer risk.* Endocr Relat Cancer. 2012 Nov 9;19(6):785-92.

Gialluria, F., et al. *Exercise training improves autonomic function and inflammatory pattern in women with polycystic ovary syndrome (PCOS).* Clin Endocrinol. 2008 Nov;69(5):792-8.

Gao, D., et al. *Interleukin-1B mediates macrophage-induced impairment of insulin signaling in human primary adipocytes..* Am J Physiol Endocrinol Metab. 2014 Aug 1;307(3):E289-304.

Garde, A., et al. *Bi-directional associations betweenpsychological arousal, cortisol, and sleep.* Behav Sleep Med. 2011 Dec 28;10(1):28-40.

Godoy-Matos, A., et al. *The potential role of increased adrenal volume in the pathophysiology of obesity-related type*

2 diabetes. J Endocrinol Invest. 2006 Feb;29(2):159-63.

Gottlieb, D., et al. *Association of sleep time with diabetes mellitus and impaired glucose tolerance.* Arch Intern Med. 2005 Apr 25;165(8):863-7.

Gunter, M., et al. *Insulin, insulin-like growth factor-1 and risk of breast cancer in postmenopausal women.* J Natl Cancer Inst. 2009 Jan 7;:101(1):48-60.

Guo, M., et al. *Metformin may produce antidepressant effects through improvement of cognitgive function among depressed patietns with diabetes mellitus.* Clin Exp Pharm Physiol. 2014 May 24.

Habib, S., et al. *Diabetes and risk of renal cell carcinoma.* J. Cancer. 2012;3:42-8.

Halloran, D. From Lectures at UW-Marshfield. 1994

Hoffman, R., et al. *Effects of glucose control and variability on endothelial function and repair in adolescents with type 1 diabetes.* ISRN Endocrin. 2013;2013:876547.

Honke, N., et al. *The p38-mediated rapid down-regulation of cell surface gp130 expression impairs interleukin-6 signaling in the synovial fluid of juvenile idiopathic arthritis patients.* Arthritis Rheumatol. 2014 Feb;66(2):470-8.

Hsu, Y., et al. *Glycated hemoglobin A1c is superior to fasting plasma glucose as an independent risk factor for colorectal neoplasia.* Cancer Causes Control. 2012 Feb;23(2):321-8.

Huang, H., et al. *Associations of green tea and rock tea consumption with risk of impaired fasting glucose and impaired glucose tolerance in Chinese men and women.* PLoS One. 2013 Nov 18;8(11):e79214.

Hussein, M., et al. *Alterations of the CD4, CD8, T cell subsets, interleukins-1B, IL-10, IL-17, tumor necrosis factor-alpha and soluble intercellular adhesion molecule-1 in rheumatoid arthritis and osteoarthritis: preliminary observations.* Pathol Oncol Res. 2008 Sep;14;(3):321-8.

Iavicoli, M., et al. *Impaired phagocytic function and increased immune complexes in diabetics with severe microangiopathy.* Diabetes. 1982 Jan;31;(1):7-11.

Imayama, I., et al. *Effects of caloric restriction weight loss diet and exercise on inflammatory biomarkers in overweight/obese postmenopausal women: a randomized controlled trial.* Cancer Res. 2012 May 1;72(9):2314-26.

Issan, Y., et al. *Elevated level of pro-inflammatory eicosanoids and EPC dysfunction in diabetic patients with cardiac ischemia.* Prost Other Lipid Mediat. 2013 Jan;100-101:15-21.

Iwamoto, T., et al. *Interleukin-21-producing c-Maf-expressing CD4 T cells induce effector DC8 T cells and enhance autoimmune inflammation in scurfy mice.* Arthritis Rheumatol. 2014 Aug;66(8):2079-90.

Jain, S., et al. *Curcumin supplementation lowers TNF-alpha, IL-6, IL-8, and MCP-1 secretion in high glucose-treated cultured monocytes and blood levels of TNF-alpha, IL-6, MCP-1, glucose, and glycosylated hemoglobin in diabetic rats.* Antioxid Redox Signal. 2009 Feb;11(2):241-9.

Jain, S., et al. *Effect of Chromium niacinate and chromium picolinate supplementation on lipid peroxidation, TNF-alpha, IL-6, CRP, glycated hemoglobin, triglycerides and cholesterol levels in blood of Streptozotocin-treated diabetic rats.* Free Radic Biol Med. 2007 Oct 15;43(8):1124-1131.

Jain, S., et al. *The effect of sleep apnea and insomnia on blood levels of leptin, insulin resistance, IP-10, and hydrogen sulfide in type 2 diabetic patients.* Metab Syndr Relat Disord. 2012 Oct;10_5):331-6.

Jolly, M., et al. *Serum free light chains, interferon-alpha, and interleukins in systemic lupus erythematosus.* Lupus. 2014 Apr 30;23(9):881-888.

Johnson, A. and Olefsky, M. *The origins and drivers of insulin resistance.* Cell. 2013. Feb 14; 152.

Joussen, A., et al. *TNF-alpha mediated apoptosis plays an important role in the development of early diabetic retinopathy and long-term histopathological alterations.* Mol. Vis. 2004; 15: 1418-1428.

Kabat, G., et al. *Repeated measures of serum glucose and insulin in relation to postmenopausal breast cancer.* Int J Cancer. 2009 Dec 1;125(11):20704-10.

Kaplar, M., et al. *The possible association of in vivio leukocyte-platelet heterophilic aggregate formation and the development of diabetic angiopathy.* Platelets. 2001 Nov;12(7):419-22.

Karahan, S., et al. *The effects of impaired trace element status on polymorphonuclear leukocyte activation in the development of vascualar complications in type 2 diabetes mellitus.* Clin Chem Lab Med. 2001 Feb;39(2):109-15.

Katon, W. *Depression and diabetes: unhealthy bedfellows.* Depress Anxiety. 2010 Apr;27(4):323-6.

Khambaty, T., et al. *Depressive symptom clusters as predictors of 6-year increaeses in insulin resistance: data from the Pittsburgh Healthy Heart Project.* Psychosom Med. 2014 Jun;76(5):363-9.

Kiechl, S., et al. *Blockade of receptor activator of nuclear factor-kB signaling improves hepatic insulin resistance and prevents development of diabetes mellitus.* Nat Med. 2013 Feb 10.

Kim, W., et al. *Prostate size correlates with fasting blood glucose in non-diabetic benign prostatic hyperplasia patients with normal testosterone levels.* J Korean Med Sci. 2011 Sep;26(9):1214-8.

Knott, R., et al. *Regluation of transforming growth factor-beta, basic fibroblast growth factor, and vascular endothelial cell growth factor mRNA in peripheral blood leukocytes in patients with diabetic retinopathy.* Metabolism. 1999 Sep;48(9):1172-8.

Krechler, T, et al. *Polymorphism -23Phl in the promoter of insulin gene and pancreatic cancer: a pilot study.* Neoplasma. 2009 56(1):26-32.

Kroenke, C., et al. *High and low fat dairy intake, recurrance, and mortality after breast cancer diagnosis.* J Natl Cancer Inst. 2013 105(9):616-623.

Krone, C. and Ely, J. *Controlling hyperglycemia as an adjunct to cancer therapy.* Integr Cancer Ther. 2005 Mar;4(1):25-31.

Kodama, M., et al. *Autoimmune disease and allergy adre controlled by vitamin C treatment.* In Vivo. 1994 Mar-Apr;8(2):251-7.

Kodama, M., et al. *Vitamin C infusion treatment enhances cortisol production of the adrenal via the pituitary ACTH route.* In Vivo. 1994 Nov-Dec;8(6):1079-85.

Kurimoto, E., et al. *IL-17 A is essential to the development of elastase-induced pulmonary inflammation and emphysema in mice.* Respir Res. 2013 Jan 20;14(1):5.

Lan, Y., et al. *The association of interleukin-21 polymorphisms with interleukin-21 serum levels and risk of systemic lupus erythematosus.* Gene. 2014 Mar 15;538(1):94-8.

Lazzeri, C., et al. *Clinical significance of glycated hemoglobin in the acute phase of ST elevation myocardial infarction.* World J Cardiol. 2014 Apr;6(4):140-147.

Lebiedz-Odrobina, D. and Kay, J. *Rheumatic manifestations of diabetes mellitus.* Rheum Dis Clin North Am. 2010 Nov;36(4):681-99.

Lee, J. and Heur, M. *Interleukin-1B enhances cell migration through Ap-K1 and NF-B pathway dependent FGF2 expression in human corneal endothelial cells.* Biol Cell. 2013 Jan 18.

Lee, S., et al. *Interleukin-17 increases the expression of Toll-like receptor 3 via th eSTAT3 pathway in rheumatoid arthritis fibroblast-like synoviocytes..* Immunology. 2014 Mar;141(3):353-61.

Leipe, J., et al. *Increased Th17 cell frequency and poor clinical outcome in rheumatoid arthritis are associated with a genetic variant in the IL4R gene, rs180510.* Arthritis Rheumatol. 2014 May;66(5):1165075.

Lenski, M. and Scherer, M. *The significance of interleukin-6 and lactate in the synovial fluid for diagnosing native septic arthritis.* Acta Orthop Belg. 2014. Mar;80(1):18-25.

Ligibel, J., et al. *Impact of mixed strength and endurance exercise intervention on insulin levels in breast cancer survivors.* J Clin Oncol. 2008 Feb 20;20;26(6):907-12.

Liu, X., et al. *The relationship between SNPs in the genes of TLR signal transduction pathway downstreatm elements and rheumatoid arthritis susceptibility*. Tsitol Genet. 2014 May-Jun;48(3):24-9.

Liu, Y., et al. *IL-1B is upregulated in the diabetic retina and retinal vessels: cell-specific effect of high glucose and IL-1B autostimulation*. PLoS One. 2012;67(5):E36949.

Ljungman, P., et al. *Modification of the interleukin-6 response of air pollution by interleukin-6 and fibrinogen polymorphisms*. Environ Health Persp. 2004 Sep. Vol 117, Issue 4:1373-1379.

Lopez-Virella, M. *Abnormal metabolism of low density lipoprotein in diabetes mellitus*. Horm Metab Res Supp. 1985;15:83-7.

Lou, J., et al. *Fasting blood glucose level and prognosis in non-small cell lung cancer patients*. Lung Cancer. 2012 May;76(2):242-7.

Lyn-Cook, B., et al. *Increased expression of toll-like receptors 7 and 9 and other cytokines in systemic lupus erythematosus patients: ethnic differences and potential new targets for therapeutic drugs*. Mol Immunol. 2014 Sep;61(1):38-43.

Ma, N., et al. *Combination of TACI-IgG and anti-IL-15 treats murine lupus by reducing mature and memory B cells*. Cell Immunol. 2014 May-Jun;289:1-2:140-4.

Magyari, L., et al. *Interleukins and interleukin receptors in rheumatoid arthritis: research, diagnostics and clinical implicaitons*. World J Orthop. 2014 Sept 18;5(4):516-36.

Malekirad, A., et al. *Neurocognitive, mental health, and glucose disorders in farmers exposed to organophosphorus pesticides*. Arh Hig Rada Toksikol. 2013;64(1):1-8.

Matejcikova, Z., et al. *Cerebrospinal fluid inflammatory markers in patients with multiple sclerosis: a pilot study*. J Neural Transm. 2014 Jun 4.

Matuszewska, A. *Mechanisms of osteoporosis development in patients with rheumatoid arthritis*. Postepy Hig Med Dosw. 2014 Feb 4;68:145-52.

Marano, C., et al. *The relationship between fasting serum glucose and cerebral glucose metabolism in late-life depression and normal aging* . Psychiatry Res. 2014 Apr 30;222(1-2):84-90.

Marhoffer, W., et al. *Impairment of polymorphonuclear leukocyte function and metabolic control of diabetes*. Diabetes Care. 1992 Feb;15(2):256-60.

Martinez, P., et al. *Impaired CD4 and T-helper 17 cell memory response to Strep Pneumonia is associated with elevated glucose and percent glycated hemoglobin A1c in Mexican Americans with type 2 diabetes mellitus*. . Transl Res. 2014 Jan;163(1):53-63.

Massin, P., et al. *Hemoglobin A1c and fasting glucose levels as predictors of retinopathy at 10 years: the French DESIR study.* Arch Opthalmol 2011 Feb;129(2):188-145.

Matthews, C., et al. *Metabolic syndrome and risk of death from cancers of the digestive system.* Metabolism. 2010 Aug;59(8):1231-9.

Mayes, T., et al. *Quantity and quality of nocturnal sleep affect morning glucose measurement in acutely burned children.* J Burn Care Res. 2013 Sep-Oct;34(5):483-91.

Memon, A., et al. *Circulating HER2 is associated with hyperglycemia and insulin resistance.* J Diabetes. 2014 Jul 1.

Mete, M., et al. *Relationship of glycemia control to lipid and blood pressure lowering and atherosclerosis: the SANDS experience.* J Diabetes Comp. 2011 Nov-Dec;25(6):362-7.

Mezuk, B., et al. *Depression, anxiety, and prevalent diabetes in the Chinese population: findings from the Cina KAdoorie Biobank of 0.5 million people.* J Psychosom Res. 2013 Dex;75(6):511-17.

Mirza, S., et al. *Type 2-diabetes is associated with elevated levels of TNF-alpha, IL-6, and adiponectin and low levels of leptin in a population of Mexican American: a cross-sectional study.* Cytokine. 2012 Jun;57(1): 136-52.

Misciagna, G., et al. *Serum frucosamine and colorectal adenomas.* Eur J Epidemiol. 2004;19(5):425-32.

Mizutuni, N., et al. *IL-33 and alveolar macrophages contribute to the mechanisms underlying the exacerbation of IgE-mediated airway inflammation and remodeling in mice.* Immunol. 2013 Jan;139(2):205-18.

Mohn, A., et al. *Persistence of impaired pancreatic beta-cell function in children treated for acute lymphoblastic leukemia.* Lancet. 2004 Jan 10;363(9403):127-8.

Motojima, K., et al. *Repetitive postprandial hypertriglyceridemia induces monocyte adhesion to aortic endothelial cells in Got-Kakizaki rats.* Endocr J. 2008 May;55:2):373-9.

Morigi, M., et al. *Leukocyte-endothelial interaction is augmented by high glucose concentrations and hyperglycemia in a NF-KB-dependent fashion.* J Clin Invest. 1998 May 1;101(9):1905-15.

Mosbah, A., et al. *Influence of serum cortisol levels on glycemic control in children with type 1 diabetes.* J Egypt Soc Parasitol. 2011 Dec;41(3):377-84.

Mullner, E., et al. *Vegetables and PURA-rich plant oil reduce DNA strand breaks in individuals with type 2 diabetes.* Mol Nutr Food Res. 2013 Feb;57(2):328-38.

Nakajima, H., et al. *Association between sleep duration and hemoglobin A1c level.* Sleep Med. 2008 Oct;9(7):745-52.

Neuhouser, M., et al. *A low-glycemic load diet reduces serum C-reactive protein and modestly increases adiponectin in overweight and obese adults.* J Nutr. 2012 Feb;142(2):369-74.

Nishimura, R., et al. *Relationship between hemoglobin A1c and cardiovascular disease in mild-to-moderated hypercholesterolemic Japanese individuals: subanalysis of a large-scale randomized controlled trial.* Cardiovasc Diabetol. 2011 June 30:10-58.

Oikawa, Y., et al. *NKT cell frequency in Japanese type 1 diabetes.* Ann NY Acad Sci. 2003 Nov;1005:230-2.

Okano, K., et al. *Exploration of hematological and immunological changes associated with the severity of type 2 diabetes mellitus in Japan.* Nurs Health Sci. 2008 Mar;10(1):65-9.

Onitilo, A. *Type 2 diabetes mellitus, glycemic control, and cancer risk.* Eur J Cancer Prev. 2014 Mar;23(2):134-40.

Ortiz, A., et al. *Insulin resistance, central obesity, and risk of colorectal adenomas.* Cancer. 2012 Apr 1;118(7):1774-81.

Osaki, Y., et al. *Metabolic syndrome and incidence of liver and breast cancers in Japan.* Cancer Epidemiol. 2012 Apr;36(2):141-7.

Ozturk, B., et al. *Effect of serum cytokines and VEGF levels on diabetic retinopathy and macular thickness.* Mol Vision. 2009 15:1906-1914.

Pan, H., et al. *Targeting T-helper 9 cells and interleukin-9 in autoimmune diseases.* Cytokine Growth Factor Rev. 2013 Dec;24(6):515-22.

Pandeya, D., et al. *Role of hyperinsulininemia in increased risk of prostate cancer: a case control study from Kathmandu Valley.* Asian Pac J Cancer Prev. 2014;15(2):1031-5.

parents.com

Park, W., et al. *Causal effects of synthetic chemicals on mitochondrial deficits and diabetes pandemic.* Arch Pharm Res. 2013 Feb;36(2):178-88.

Parlapiano, C., et al. *The relationship between glycated hemoglobin and polymorphonuclear leukocyte leukotriente B4 release in people with diabetec mellitus.* Diabetes Res Clin Pract. 1999 Oct;46(1):43-5.

pathwaycommons.org

Pereria, C., et al. *DNA damage and cytotoxicity in adult subjects with prediabetes.* Mutat Res. 2013 May 15;753(2):76-81.

Percival, S., et al. *Bioavailability of herbs and spices in humans as determined by ex vivo inflammatory suppression and DNA strand breaks.* J Am Coll Nutr. 2012 Aug;31(4):288-94.

Pfeiler, G., et al. *Influence of insulin resistance on adiponectin receptor expression in breast cancer.* Maturitas. 2009

Jul 20;63(3):253-6.

Piatkiewicz, P., et al. *The dysfunction of NK cells in patients with type 2 diabetes and colon cancer.* Arch Immunol Ther Exp. 2013 June;61(3):245-53.

Priou, P., et al. *Independent association between obstructive sleep apnea severity and glycated hemoglobin in adults without diabetes.* Diabetes Care. 2012 Sep;35(9):1902-6.

Profumo, E., et al. *T lymphocyte autoreactivity in inflammatory mechanisms regulating atherosclerosis.* Sci Wld Jrl. 2012;157534.

Pyykkonen, A., et al. *Sleep duration and insulin resistance in individuals without type 2 diabettes: the PPP-botnia study.* Ann Med. 2014 May 9.

Rafraf, M., et al. *Omega-e acids improve glucose metabolism without effects on obesity values and serum visfatin levels in women with polycystic ovary syndrome.* J Am Coll Nutr. 2012 Oct;31(5):361-8.

Reynolds, R., et al. *Elevated fasting plasma cortisol is associated with ischemic heart disease and its risk factors in people with type 2 diabetes: the Edinburgh type 2 diabetes study.* J Clin Endocrinol Metab. 2010 Apr;95(4):1602-8.

Richens, E., et al. *T-lymphocyte subpopulations in type 1 diabetes mellitus. A longitudinal study.* Acta Diabetol Lat. 1985 Jul-Sep;22(3):299-38.

Rodenbeck, A., et al. *Interactions between evening and nocturnal cortisol secretion and sleep parameters in patietns with sever chronic primary insomnia.* Neurosci Lett. 2002 May 17;324(2):159-63.

Rossi, S., et al. *Cerebrospinal fluid detection of interleukin-1B in phase of remisison predicts disease progression in multiple sclerosis.* J Neuroinflammation. 2014 Feb 18;11:32.

Rubolf, S., et al. *Elevated IL-6 levels in patients with atypical depression but not in patients with typical depression.* Psychiatry Res. 2014 Jun 30;217(1-2):34-8.

Safdie, F., et al. *Fasting enhances the response of glioma to chemo-and radiotherapy.* PloS One. 2012;7(9):e44603.

Saha, S., et al. *Circulating very-low-density lipoprotein from subjects with impaired glucose tolerance accelerates adrenocortical cortisol and aldosterone synthesis.* Horm Metab Res. 2013 Feb;45(2):169-72.

Sanchez, P., et al. *Prevalence of diabetes in a cancer population in a Malaga hospital.* Nutr Hosp. 2012 Mar-Apr;27(2):456-62.

Sasaki, H., et al. *Prevalence and risk factors for erectile dysfunction in Japanese diabetics.* Diabetes Res Clin Pract. 2005 Oct;70(1):81-9.

Scnm.edu alumni association posting on 2014 Dec 19 from marketing@scnm.edu.

Selvin, E., et al. *Glycated hemoglobin, diabetes, and cardiovascular risk in nondiabetic adults.* N Engl J Med. 2010 Mar;362(9):800-11.

Seppi, D., et al. *Cerebrospinal fluid IL-1B correlates with cortical pathology load in multiple sclerosis at clinical onset.* JNeuroimmunology. 2014 May 15;270(1-2):56-60.

Seyfried, T. *Cancer as a metabolic disease: implications for novel therapeutics.* Presentation at the OncANP conference, July 2013.

Sieri, S., et al. *Prospective study on the role of glucose metabolism in breast cancer occurrence.* Int J Cancer. 2012 Feb 15;130(4):921-9.

Singh, A., et al. *Relation of glycated hemoglobin with carotid atherosclerosis in ischemic stroke patients: an observational study in Indian population.* Annals of Indian Academy of Neru. 2013 Apr-Jun;16(2):185-189.

Sjogren, A., et al. *Magnesium deficiency in IDDM related to level of glycosylated hemoglobin.* Diabetes. 1986 Apr;35(4):459-63.

Skoczen, S., et al. *Markers of metabolic syndrome and peptides regulating metabolism in survivors of childhood acute lymphoblastic leukemia.* Przegl Lek. 2011;68(9):592-6.

sueden.com

Skwarecki, B. *Artificial sweeteners linked to glucose intolerance.* www.medscape.com. 2014 Sept 17.

Shamhart, P., et al. *Hyperglycemia enhances function and differentiation of adult rat cardiac fibroblasts.* Can J Physiol Pharmacol. 2014 Jul;92(7):598-604.

Sharhar, S., et al. *Anitoxidant intake and status, and oxidative stress in relation to breast cancer risk: a case-control study.* Asian Pac J Cancer Prev. 2008 Apr-Jun;9(2):343-49.

Shu, C., et al. *The immune system's involvement in obesity-driven type 2 diabetes.* Semin Immunol. 2013 Jan 17.

Smith, J. and Colbert, R. *Review: the interleukin-23/interleukin-17 axis in spondyloarthritis pathogenesis Th17 and beyond.* Arthritis Rheumatol. 2014 Feb;66(2):231-41.

Snell-Bergeon, J., et al. *Inflammatory markers are increased in youth with type 1 diabetes: the SEARCH case-control study.* J Clin Endocrinol Metab. 2010 June;95(6):2888-2876.

sonnetskitchen.com

Soranzo, N. *Genetic determinants of variability in glycated hemoglobin a1c in humans: review of recent progress and prospects for use in diabetes care.* Curr Diab Rep. 2011 Dec;11(6):562-569.

Soromou, L., et al. *Astragalin attenuates lipopolysaccharide-induced inflammatory responses by down-regulating NF-kB signaling pathway.* Biochem Biophys Res Commun. 2012 Mar 9;419(2):256-61.

Soumaya, K. *Molecular mechanisms of insulin resistance in diabetes.* Adv Exp Med Biol. 2012;771:240-51.

Stattin, P., et al. *Prospective study of hyperglycemia and cancer risk.* Diabetes Care. 2007 Mar;30(3):561-7.

Stevens, E., et al. *Hemoglobin A1c and the relationship to stage and grade of endometrial cancer.* Arch Gynecol Obstet. 2012 Dec;286(6):1507-12.

Strom, A., et al. *Pronounced reduction of cutaneous Langerhans cell density in recently diagnosed type 2 diabetes.* Diabetes. 2014 Mar;63(3):1148-53.

Sudo, C., et al. *Clinical significance of neutrophil apoptosis in peripheral blood of patients with type 2 diabetes mellitus.* Lab Hematol. 2007;13(3):108-12.

Surendar, J., et al. *Increased levels of both Th1 and Th2 cytokines in subjects with metabolic syndrome (CURES-103).* Diabetes Technol Ther. 2011 Apr;13(4):477-82.

Teno, S., et al. *Increased activity of membrane glycoprotein PC-1 in the fibroblasts from non-insulin-dependent diabetes mellitus patients with insulin resistance.* Diabetes Res Clin Pract. 1999 Aug;45(1):35-30.

Teran-perez, G., et al. *Steroid hormones and sleep regulation.* Mini Rev Med Chem. 2012 Oct;12(11):1040-8.

Trenova, A., et al. *Cytokines and disability in interferon-b-1b treated and untreated women with multiple sclerosis.* Arch Med Res. 2014 Aug;45(6):495-500.

Udell, E. 1994. Lectures from SCNM, Tempe, AZ.

USDA.gov

Uygur-Bayramicili, O., et al. *Type 2 diabetes mellitus and CA 19-9 levels.* World J Gastroenterol. 2007 Oct 28;13(40):5357-9.

Valcamonica, E., et al. *Levels of Il-8 in the synovial fluid of patients with inflammatory arthritides and osteoarthritis.* Clin Exp Rheumatol. 2014 Mar-Apr;32(2):243-50.

Van der Geest, K., et al. *Disturbed B cell homeostasis in newly diagnosed giant cell arteritis and polymyalgia rheumatica.* Arthritis Rheumatol. 2014 Jul;66(7):1927-38.

Van de Weijer, T., et al. *Relationships between mitochondrial function and metabolic flexibility in type 2 diabetes mellitus.* PLoS One. 2013;8(2):e51648.

Varga, T., et al. *Higher serum DPP-4 enzyme activity and decreased lymphocyte CCD26 expression in type 1 diabetes.* Pathol Oncol Res. 2011 Dec;17(4):925-30.

Vasisht, K., et al. *Differences in insulin secretion and sensitivity in short-sleep insomnia.* Sleep. 2013 Jun 1;36(6):955-7.

Vgontzas, A., et al. *Insomnia with objective short sleep duration is associated with type 2 diabetes: a population-based study.* Diabetes Care. 2009 Nov;32(11):1980-5.

Vgontzas, A., et al. *Chronic insomnia is associated with nyctohemeral activation fo the hypothalamic-pituitary-adrenal axis: clinical implications.* J Clin Endocrinol Metab. 2001 Aug;86(8):3787-94.

Vgontzas, A., et al. *IL-6 and its circadian secreation in humans.* Neuroimmunomodulation. 2005;12(3):131-40.

Wada, T., et al. *Aberrant histone acetylation contributes to elevated interleukin-6 production in rheumatoid arthritis synovial fibroblasts.* Biochem Biophys Res Commun. 2014 Feb 21;444(4):682-6.

Waggiallah, H. and Alzohairy, M. *The effect of oxidative stress on human red cells glutathione peroxidase, glutathione redeuctase levels, and prevalence of anemia among diabetics.* N Am J Med Sci. 2011 July;63(7):344-347.

webmd.com

Weltin, A. and Lavin, R. *The effect of a community garden on HgA1c in diabetics of Marshallese descent.* J. Community Health Nurs. 2012 Jan;29(1):12-24.

Woolf, E., et al. *The ketogenic diet for the treatment of malignant glioma.* J Lipid Res. 2014 Feb 6.

Wright, E., et al. *Oxidative stress in type 2 diabetes: the role of fasting and postprandial glycaemia.* Int J Clin Pract. 2006 mar;60(3): 308-314.

Wu, Q., et al. *Metabolic syndrome components and risk factors for pancreatic adenocarcinoma: a case-control study in China.* Digestion. 2012;86(4):294-301.

Yang, Y., et al. *Serial glycosylated hemoglobin levels and risk of colorectal neoplasia among patietns with type 2 diabetes mellitus.* Cancer Epidemiol Biomarkers Prev. 2010 Dec; 19(12):3027-3036.s

Yasunari, K., et al. *Oxidativae stress in leukocytes is a possible link between blood pressure, blood glucose, and C-reacting protein.* Hypertension. 2002 Mar 1;39(3):777-80.

Yue, W., et al. *Impact of glycemic control on circulating endothelial progenitor celsl and arterial stiffness in patients with type 2 diabetes mellitus.* Cardiovasc Diabetol. 2011 Dec 20;10:113.

Xuan, Y., et al. *High-glucose inhibits human fibroblast cell migration in wound healing via repression of bFGF-regulating JNK phosphorylation.* PLOS. 2014 Sep;10.1371.

Xiao, Y., et al. *TPL2 mediates autoimmune inflammation through activation of the TAK! Axis of IL-17 signaling.* J Exp Med. 2014 Jul 28;211(8):1689-702.

Zhao, L., et al. *Immunoregulation therapy changes the frequency of interleukin-22 CD4 P cells in systemic lupus erythematosus.* Clin exp Innunol. 2014 Jul;177(1):212-8.

Zhou, H., et al. *Diabetes, prediabetes and cancer mortality.* Diabetogia. 2010 Sep;53(9):1867-76.

Zhou, H., et al. *Determinants of leukocyte adenosine triphosphate-binding cassette transporter G1 gene expression in type 2 diabetes mellitus.* Metabolism. 2008 Aug;57(8):1135-40.

Zieman, S., et al. *Hemoglobin A1c and arterial and ventricular stiffness in older adult.* PLoS One. 2012; 7(10):e4791.

Zenaro, E., et al. *Use of imaging to study leukocyte trafficking in the central nervous system.* Immunol Cell Biol. 2013 Jan22.

www.ingramcontent.com/pod-product-compliance
Lightning Source LLC
Chambersburg PA
CBHW041605260326

41914CB00012B/1394